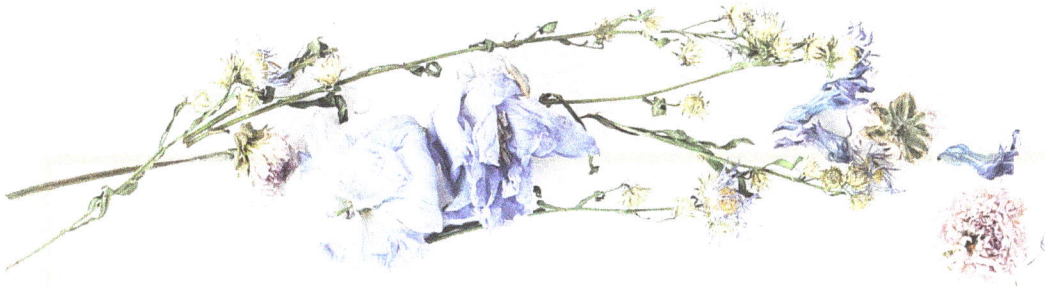

BEYOND *Beauty*

A Guide for Beautiful Skin and Creating Your Own Homemade Products

by BETHEL JIRICEK

Green Eyed Grace LLC

Greeley, Colorado

Green Eyed Grace LLC
Greeley, CO 80634
© 2019 Bethel Jiricek

Published 2019

Cover design and book layout by Mindy Stephens Creative
Illustrations © 2019 Bethel Jirecek
Cover images and photos from Adobe Stock

ISBN 978-1-7342255-0-1

This book is dedicated to my beautiful children:
Anthony, Jorey, Tyler and Grace.

"The Lord bless you and keep you; the
Lord make his face to shine upon you and
be gracious to you; the Lord lift up his
countenance upon you and give you peace."

Numbers 6:24-26

A special thank you to my husband, Jeremy, for supporting me
through the long process of writing a book and standing by my
side as I grow and do crazy things. I love you more than you know.

I would also like to thank my beautiful sister, Rachelle,
for always supporting me and being a light in the darkness.

And finally, I would like to thank Amy for her inspiration,
keeping the business afloat and her continued encouragement.

TABLE OF CONTENTS

Introduction: HOW I BECAME A NATURAL SKIN-CARE ADVOCATE

Over the years, I have developed a strong passion for finding products that are free of chemicals, have minimal ingredients, and that are beneficial for the skin. In fact, I have such a passion for clean skin care that I created the Green Eyed Grace product line. Having my own skin-care line allows me to offer cleaner products with natural and organic ingredients to family, friends, and clients. When I was a teenager, the idea of proper skin care was the last thing on my mind. That was a luxury I could not afford. Often a person, especially a teenager, cannot afford high-end professional skin-care products—or any luxury-type products for that matter.

When I was a teen, my mom did not have much money. I lived with her and my younger sister in a little-bitty trailer on the outskirts of a town in Northern Colorado. My mom was a single mother of four children, who worked as a waitress and attended college, with a dream to become a teacher. Although I visited my dad quite often, my love of beauty products really originated at my mother's home.

I don't have many memories of shopping other than for minimal groceries, and we bought the cheapest things we could find. Cutting coupons, especially for groceries, and watching for sale items was expected. We bought almost all of our personal-care products at the grocery store or local drugstore. The most expensive beauty product I ever purchased as a teen was a foundation from Mary Kay, which was considered "high-end" in my family. I remember saving my allowance for weeks so that I could buy this makeup. However, I would have never thought of saving my allowance for a cleanser or moisturizer! That was just a cheap drugstore purchase if we splurged. The cheaper the better, was our motto.

My obsession with skin care and makeup was ignited when my mom received a used Mary Kay kit from one of her friends. The pink-vinyl suitcase was packed full of samples. It had tons of tiny little lipsticks, blush in every color, little vials of cleansers, and a miniature blue toner that smelled so pretty. I clung to the suitcase, begging my Mom to let me use it. Thankfully she was not as impressed with the pink suitcase as I was. I spent days going over every item. I tried every single product in it. Even the dark, purplish brown lipstick. Unbeknownst to me at the time, my sweet little sister was my very first client. And thankfully she was a willing participant.

As I grew into an adult, my love for beauty products only grew stronger. I loved playing with color and searching through magazines for different makeup styles. I would clip out my favorite looks and put them in a binder, just in case I wanted to refer to them later. My binder was organized by parts of the face, such as eyes and cheeks. I still look through that binder from time to time.

I originally thought I would be a makeup artist but was sorely disappointed to find it was not a fulfilling job position for my personality. Many of the women who hired me wanted a quick "face" put on. There was no concern about the ingredients in the makeup or their quality. In fact, most of them wanted to completely cover their natural beauty. They requested airbrushed, heavy makeup that was far from natural. Because of my past experience with building my own confidence and self-esteem, this did not sit well with me. I have learned— the hard way—that makeup should only be used to enhance beauty, not conceal it.

Coats of makeup never look natural. I learned this lesson after I spent many years wearing heavy makeup. It was my way of hiding from myself and the world. During those years, I struggled the most and felt worse about myself than ever before. I attracted the wrong people into my life because I felt so down on myself. I had convinced myself that I was ugly and too different from everyone. I had super-fair skin, which led to a very uneven skin tone. I did not have the confidence to know that just because I was different did not mean that I was not beautiful. That is why you will find a chapter on confidence in this book. It really does go hand in hand with beauty.

The same mentality can be true for skin-care products. Way too often in my profession, I see salons and spas shouting out specials for chemical peels, micro-blading or micro-needling in order to look "young" again. So many harsh treatments are being encouraged and used in order to have younger looking skin, when in reality beautiful skin comes from pampering it and long-term healthy routines, such as eating nutritious foods. (See chapter 18 for more about eating right for your skin.)

For those who watch their budget closely, receiving spa treatments or even spa products may not be feasible, and in my opinion these harsh treatments or products are rarely worth the cost. Even though some of us cannot afford these luxuries, it does *not* mean we should compromise on what we use on our skin. Cheap, drugstore products often contain very harsh chemicals that can hurt the skin and might even be harmful to the body as well since our skin absorbs the products we apply.

"Never let money get in the way of taking care of yourself."

—Bethel Jiricek

I discovered my true desire to make my own healthy skin-care products when my youngest son was struggling with eczema. He was about two years old when he had a severe eczema outbreak, and I rushed him to the doctor, worried he had an allergic reaction to something. Our family doctor at the time informed us it was "only eczema" that was caused by the heat of summer. She then recommended we leave our small child in wet pajamas for a couple hours for the next two nights. She prescribed a cortisone cream and sent us on our way. Thankfully, I never followed her recommendation on the wet jammies—in fact, I would *never* recommend anyone dress their toddler in wet PJs for any amount of time.

Although the cortisone cream began to clear up my son's outbreak, it lingered and continued to return and subside for several more years. I spoke with a few professionals in the holistic-health field who recommended we change my son's diet, skin-care products, and our household cleaning products. I began making my own laundry detergent and creams to help his skin. I also finally understood that certain foods were my son's primary problem. With all these adjustments in lifestyle, we began seeing long-term, positive changes by the time he was five.

As a skin-care specialist, I was constantly testing lotions, soaps, and skin-care-type products sold at stores. I was shocked to discover how many harmful ingredients they contained. We *really* have to be our own advocates and protect our families from the toxic chemicals we are exposed to every day. Many of us feel consumed by the time and effort it takes to choose healthy products, not to mention the financial cost of higher-end lotions, serums, and creams.

It took almost a year for my son's eczema to improve from the combination of an anti-allergenic diet and my homemade detergents and lotions, but I was greatly encouraged that I was able to bring him relief. I also wanted to help other families benefit from cleaner skin-care products, so

I began sharing my recipes with family, friends, and on my blog (www.GreenEyedGrace.com).

A big part of my passion as a mom and a skin-care expert is to empower people to create budget-friendly and skin-friendly personal-care products. That is why I decided to write this book: to share what I've learned with anyone interested in healthy skin.

Even if you are on a strict budget, you can use the recipes in this book to make luxury items at home that will make your skin feel like you just had a professional skin treatment. They can be as simple or as complex as you like. A gentle, homemade facial mask or scrub can give your skin an instant glow. Additionally, consistent healthy eating can help your skin long term. Because food plays such an important role in skin care, I included healthy smoothie recipes in chapter 18 for you to enjoy.

When you purchase the ingredients you need in the recipes, keep the overall quality of your final product in mind. I buy as many organic ingredients as I can, so that my final product will be as pure as possible and free of synthetic fertilizers and pesticides. I am a firm believer in organic ingredients because they are better for your overall health. All recipes can be made with organic ingredients, which will result in a higher quality product for your skin.

All the recipes I've assembled in this book allow for creativity, which is one of the biggest blessings we could ever ask for. Do not be afraid to try different beneficial ingredients or swap out ingredients that do not work for you or your skin type. Always tailor your skin-care line to your specific needs.

Be your own skin-care specialist. Enjoy the process of owning it *and* making it yourself.

"Creativity is the way I share
my soul with the world."

—Brené Brown

CHAPTER 1

Self-Confidence:

A MIND-BODY MAKEOVER

Why include a chapter on confidence in a DIY skin-care book? Well, let me explain. Confidence has been such a huge part of my self-growth. I could not write this book without sneaking in a few things I have learned along the way. We can have all the products or luxuries at our fingertips, but they mean *absolutely nothing* if we are miserable inside or are not able to truly appreciate them.

The cycle of self-loathing is linked to a cycle of self-neglect. When we feel bad about ourselves, we tend to look bad because we begin to neglect ourselves. Not looking our best makes us feel worse about ourselves. And the downward spiral begins. I have found that a habit of self-care can promote a healthy cycle of self-respect. Self-respect boosts our confidence.

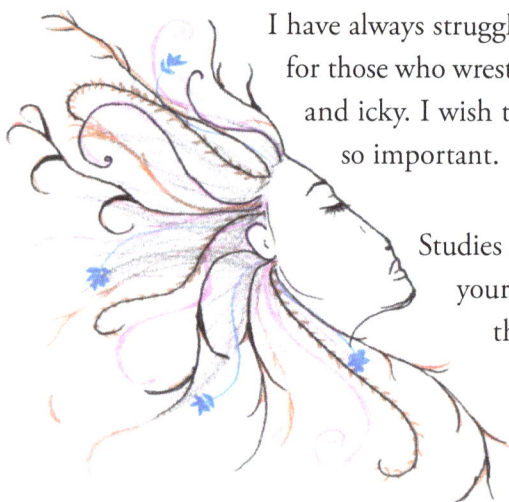

I have always struggled to feel confident in myself, so I have empathy for those who wrestle with *self-love*. The word alone just sounds weird and icky. I wish there were a better word for self-love because it *is* so important.

Studies have shown that taking care of yourself, especially your physical appearance, can lead to greater success in the working world. Those who take time for themselves and strive to learn and grow from personal challenges advance much further in life and in their careers. The key to self-confidence is to look inside yourself. The next step is to take care of yourself and set life goals. Sounds so simple, I know. However, this is a great challenge.

Pocahontas was a gentle, yet confident, person who stood firm in her beliefs.

Socrates may not have been the first to say, "Know thyself," but he's well known for the phrase. Many wise men (and women) have emphasized this simple saying. Socrates takes it a little further by saying, "The unexamined life is not worth living."

Carl Gustav Jung, who basically founded analytical psychology, stressed the importance of trying to know yourself, understanding that you are not alone, and the importance of spending time thinking on greater things. I love his quote from *The Red Book*: "Scholarliness alone is not enough; there is a knowledge of the heart that gives deeper insight. The knowledge of the heart is in no book and is not to be found in the mouth of any teacher, but grows out of you like the green seed from the dark earth."

Usually when someone says you need to "get to know yourself" it can leave a person feeling at a loss about what to do. We usually think we know ourselves pretty darn well since we spend every single day with ourselves. Surprisingly this is not the case. Many will not spend time thinking of themselves because it feels selfish or superficial.

Even though this may seem like a noble approach, those who refuse to look at themselves may end up focusing on other people or objects in an unhealthy way. For example, a man obsessed with financial success who hyper-focuses on work might not notice that his health is failing or that his family is neglected. Or, consider the hard-working, stay-at-home mom who focuses so much on her children's sports schedules and school activities that she completely neglects her own needs.

When I was younger, I really focused on what I thought other people expected of me and tried to act the way I thought they wanted me to act. I did not want to look at myself or try to discover who I really was inside. I did not like that I was so scared and shy around people. For years I tried to be the life of the party, always showing up and being "on." I was totally miserable and no longer liked who I was. Even though, at the time, I was trying to be someone I *really* thought I wanted to be, it is just *not* who I was. I now fully accept myself as an introvert and am patient with myself when I need a break.

So how do we get to know ourselves better? One good place to start your self-assessment is personality testing. Some personality types *love* this idea, while others are put off by it because they do not want to be placed in a box or told who they are. If you are the latter, stay with me! I like to look at personalities objectively, as a tool for understanding oneself not as black and white. The great thing about learning more about yourself is that if you do not like something, you can work on improvement or acceptance.

My favorite personality test is the Myers-Briggs Type Indicator (MBTI) test that discusses the 16 different personalities. This is the test that really helped me understand my quirky ways. I am an INFJ on the Myers Briggs typing model. That means that I am introverted (I), intuitive (N), feeling (F) and judging (J). Each letter represents a little about your personality. Learning about my personality really helped me understand myself AND others better. I can now really appreciate why extroverts need people, thinkers need facts, feelers need to express themselves and so on. Visit myersbriggs.org or 16personalities.com to discover your own personality type.

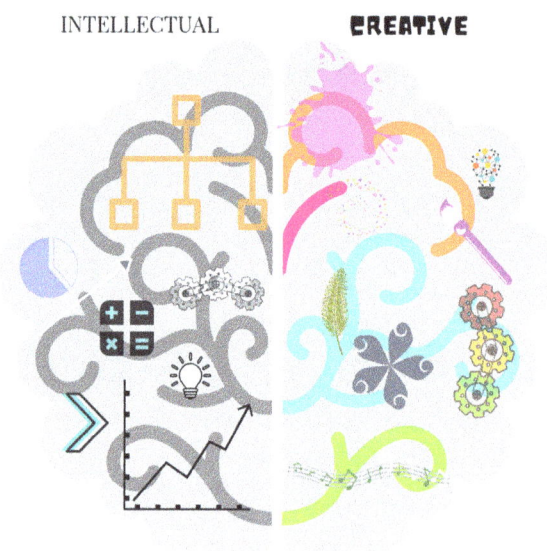

INTELLECTUAL   CREATIVE

Left brain = analytical. Right brain = creative.

A different way to discover your personality is by using the right brain/left brain test. Some people love facts, logic, and strategy (left-brain dominant), while others love creativity, energy, and ideas (right-brain dominant). And some people possess a beautiful combination of both right and left-brained traits. Certain people enjoy a lot of conversation, and others like to be quiet. Neuropsychologist Roger W. Sperry discovered the right-brain versus left-brain distinctions in the 1960s. However, there are many online tests to help you determine your dominant side. I prefer the free resource at PersonalityMax.com. This may seem very basic, but for those who have never really looked inside their heart, it can be pretty overwhelming to finally get to know yourself.

A great way to look at your own heart is to ask *why* you like and dislike certain things. Sometimes we do not like a particular thing because we associate it with a bad experience. When we are forced to look at those bad experiences, we can heal from them. This kind of assessment might actually end up with you liking that previously disliked thing after all.

We live in a very self-focused world, and many people suffer as a result of self-absorption and neglect. **However, being selfish is different from taking care of yourself.** A morning routine that includes putting on makeup, brushing your hair, or your preferred grooming method is *not* vanity unless you are obsessed with it. Taking time to organize your thoughts and drink a vitamin-packed smoothie are healthy choices, not selfish. When we take care of ourselves, we are showing ourselves, our children, and our loved ones that we matter. By doing this we are modeling to them that they matter too.

Keeping a tidy appearance boosts your self-esteem. When you feel good about yourself, you attract healthy people into your life, and you become a positive influence on those around you, including your family. When your children, spouse, sister, or mother see that you have more confidence, it encourages them to do the same.

Practicing self-care can also improve job performance and help you excel in your profession. Well-run companies look for employees who take care of themselves because it shows them that you can also take care of your role in their company.

It is easy to give up on self-care when we feel down about ourselves. Sometimes the last thing we want to do is get all dolled up for no reason. But self-care has amazing power. Negativity can be powerful as well, which is why it is so important to avoid it. What messages are you sending to yourself on a daily basis? If your thoughts are not mostly positive, it may be time to make some changes.

Self-talk or affirmations can really help improve self-confidence. We unknowingly tell ourselves many negative things throughout the day, such as "How could I be such a screw-up?" or "I could never accomplish that." Instead, consistently tell yourself positive things such as "I forgive that person" or "I am happy with my choices" or "I love my job." Always try to see the positive, even when you are feeling down. Thinking positive thoughts can often pull you out of negativity.

I'm an expert at stepping into the quicksand of negativity. I often have to check in with myself to stay positive. It is so important to avoid getting down on yourself by listening to negative self-talk or internalizing the mean, insensitive things you may have heard when you were a child—or even as an adult.

I can relate to feeling hurt by criticism during my childhood. I was a red-headed, freckle-faced kid who was teased relentlessly in grade school and beyond. I was super-awkward, underweight, and timid for most of my preteen and teen years. To add to it, I was also a highly sensitive soul who internalized most of my true feelings.

Are the words in your head mostly positive?

I felt so alone going through the rough insecurity of my adolescence. Surprisingly, so many of us felt or continue to feel this way! We all have vulnerable times of feeling inadequate, unattractive, and an outcast from society, and some of us deeply internalize these hurts because we are more sensitive than others. However, there is still some commonality in our wandering growth from childhood to adulthood.

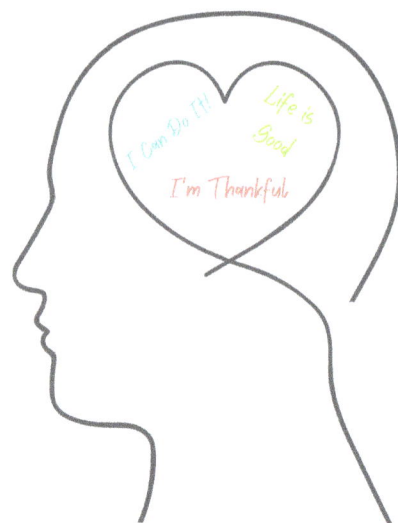

> "You are altogether beautiful, my darling; there is no flaw in you."

—Song of Solomon 4:7

Lack of confidence can hinder how we feel about our appearance. It can also prevent us from being who we are truly meant to be in the world—whether that is a baker, a lawyer, or a stay-at-home mother. Having the confidence to let others see the light that shines through you is a beautiful thing. Matthew 5:15 says, "Neither do men light a candle and put it under a bushel, but on a candlestick; and it giveth light unto all that are in the house." Letting your light shine in the world can include trying new things such as the do-it-yourself recipes in this book or sharing your unique gifts with the world.

CONFIDENTLY CREATING
NATURAL SKIN-CARE PRODUCTS

In this book, I want to empower you to make healthy, non-toxic skin-care and beauty products for yourself and your family. That said, getting the hang of DIY recipes takes a little patience and can be challenging. Sometimes recipes do not work out the way you expect. Sometimes you forget an ingredient or try to substitute an oil, and the concoction turns out horrible. Often you are trying to save money and end up spending it on experiments that may not turn out the first time or two!

If you are wondering why a recipe did not turn out as planned, please understand that I have been there. Thankfully, the recipes in this book have all been tested numerous times. Before they made it to the book, they were altered several times and some were ditched. The ones that made the grade, however, were absolutely loved. I have tried my hardest to make sure every recipe included will give you great results. However, things can still go wrong and cause frustration. Hang in there, my friend.

I can honestly share with you that it took me an entire, painstaking year to figure out how to make lotion. I tried every do-it-yourself recipe I could find. I even bought books on how to make lotion, which apparently is some sort of mystery concoction that no one is able to make at home. Most of the lotion recipes available in the books I purchased either gave the same result as the online DIY recipes or were full of bad chemicals that I had to buy at a lab. I started to number my recipes so I could keep track of the latest batch. It actually became a joke around my house: "What number are you working on now?" One failed version of Lavender/Calendula Nourishing Body Lotion became known as "Lotion No. 38."

I literally went through hundreds of lotion recipes before I was happy with one. Along the way, I had lotion separate, curdle, harden, stink, mold—you name it! I wanted to give up so many times, but something inside me could not let it go. Succeeding was everything to me because my son needed a lotion that did not irritate his skin. I was determined to figure it out. Do you know what number it was before my lotion concoction actually worked? It was number eighty-six. Yep, eighty-six times until I had a lotion I could even use. I have not shared that recipe because it turns out that particular lotion is quite complex. So I'm saving it for a different book! I have, however, included some amazing body butter recipes that are much easier and fun to make.

I have learned many things through the process of perfecting DIY skin-care recipes and creating a natural and organic skin-care line. Both experiences have definitely boosted my confidence. The more failures you have, the more likely you will have success. The more positive thoughts you have, the more likely you will be happy and successful. But most importantly, I learned that prayer will bring you through any trial you face in life. Having a strong faith has boosted my confidence more than anything else.

"Every true and perfect gift comes from above."

—James 1:17

The good Lord does not mind if you pray about what your family needs or if you ask for help with making a product or food to help heal them. Prayer is my true secret to success. I needed a solution to help my son, so I prayed and prayed. God helped me find my true passion and use it for a solution. And He will help you find yours as well.

CHAPTER 2

The Beauty of Making

YOUR OWN PRODUCTS

My rule of thumb is that if you cannot understand the ingredients listed on the back of your product, they are probably not good for your skin. Often there are about twenty ingredients listed with names we cannot pronounce, and most of them were synthesized in a laboratory. I like to keep skin care simple with ingredients you can understand. Even though lotion and personal-care products have changed over the last few decades, I *do* believe we can get back to quality products. We should take pride in our products and appreciate them as a luxury.

Making your own products can be extremely fulfilling. Taking your beauty and health needs into your own hands and tailoring products to your exact needs is powerful and life changing. We don't need mega-corporations to charge a fortune for skin-care products we may not even need.

"He has made everything beautiful in its time."

—Ecclesiastes 3:11

THE QUALITY OF MANUFACTURED PERSONAL-CARE PRODUCTS

Has the integrity of our products been lost? That was the question on my mind when I was immersed in lotion making. I truly wanted to understand how lotion was originally made and how it had changed over time. While researching and looking back through history, I could not help but feel skin-care products have lost integrity. Although harmful ingredients are not a really a new thing, they appear to be the norm now.

In Ancient Rome, women used white lead (also called "cerussa") to lighten their faces. The lead was highly toxic to their skin and bodies. Even though many Romans knew the effects of lead on their body, they insisted on using the white face powder. For many, having a lightened complexion was more important than the consequences. This sounds a little like what is happening with our products today.

Although there were a few exceptions, like lead in face powder, most remedies in the past were very natural. Oils, herbs, honey, and even milk were widely used by women—and men—for cosmetic purposes. Milk softened the skin while herbs brightened, calmed, or nourished the skin. Most products contained natural and healing ingredients. However, over time, more and more harmful ingredients have appeared.

The 1800s

I believe that most manufacturers start out with good intentions. However, eventually they begin to turn to the best "quick-fix" products for the best revenue. For example, Pond's Cold Cream started out as a medicine company in the mid-1800s. Their original beauty product was Pond's Extract, which today would have been considered a nice toner for our skin. However they were using it to treat all kinds of skin issues, mostly scrapes and minor injuries.

In 1914 the company began advertising Pond's Cold Cream, and it evolved from there. Pond's may have been the first company to encourage the "facial system" by insisting that ladies need two creams. This is funny, because now we all use about six different products on our faces! Typical facial systems now consist of cleanser, toner, moisturizer, serums, eye cream, and occasionally a facial mask. It was much simpler in the past!

The 1900s

Elizabeth Arden's skin-care products were popular in the early 1900s. Ms. Arden also had a great deal to do with facial systems. Well known for teaching proper makeup application, Ms. Arden was ahead of her time with her scientific formulas for cosmetics. She prided herself on using the products in a ladylike fashion and maintaining a classy appearance. Ms. Arden was successful in preserving that appearance. Her company has a highly influential presence to this day.

Sustainability

One thing I love about making my own products is the feeling of sustainability. If there is ever a time when you cannot make it to the grocery store or there is some disaster that disrupts our ability to buy things at a store, it is comforting to know that we can make do for a while on our own. Besides, making your own products gives you so much room for creativity. Once you learn the basics of the DIY recipes, they will also save you money. Ultimately, my absolute favorite reason for making products is the fact that your skin-care ingredients will be healthier because you most likely will not be using any preservatives and are making them fresh.

Most of my recipes have a short shelf life because they contain no preservatives. Below are my best tips for preserving homemade products. You could also do some research on how to include professional preservatives if you want to extend the shelf life of your homemade products.

6 TIPS FOR PRESERVING YOUR PRODUCTS

1. Keep everything sterile. You will always want to make sure all utensils, pots, pans, and anything else you are using to prepare a recipe have been properly washed and sterilized in your dishwasher. A natural sanitizing spray is an extra precaution. (See the recipe for Fresh-Lemon Surface Sterilizer on page 19.) All countertops and containers also should be sterilized with a natural cleaner before starting. (I do not use bleach as it can be extremely harmful to your health. Instead I prefer grain alcohol and essential oils for cleaning.)

2. Leave out the water. Products with high water content can mold or turn rancid much faster than those that are oil based. Using aloe vera is a great substitute. Even though it does naturally contain water, it is better than using straight water. Not only that, but aloe and oils are also more nourishing for the skin. If you do need to use water in a recipe, be sure to use distilled or cooled, boiled water to reduce any existing contamination or bacteria.

3. Use natural preservatives. By using natural preservatives such as glycerin, colloidal silver, vitamin E, and rosemary, you will prolong the product's shelf life. The amazing thing about some natural preservatives is that they are often great for your skin. For example, colloidal silver naturally helps prevent bacterial growth and is also wonderful at repairing damaged skin and killing bacteria on your skin, that can be present in acne breakouts.

4. Use alcohol. Using grain alcohol, vodka, or rum in your recipes can help balance a product and act as a disinfectant. Additionally, alcohol has a way of carrying scent. Consequently, if you are making a perfume or deodorizer, you will smell your essential oils much better when mixed with alcohol instead of water.

5. Let it cool completely. Anytime you heat products, you should let them cool completely before you seal them in their containers. Sealing them too early can create condensation inside the container, which can lead to premature molding or bacteria. Additionally, when they are ready to be closed up, give them a little shake (if they are not in solid form) so that your product coats the entire inside of the container. This helps keep it fresh longer, especially if your product contains a natural preservative.

6. Store products properly. Knowing when to discard your homemade product is key. Do *not* keep a product if there is a weird smell or the ingredients are separating. Products that have turned can be bad for your health and skin. Date and label all products so you know when to discard them. Sometimes products can turn before you expected because an ingredient was not quite pure or the product became too hot or cold and caused it to break down. When in doubt, throw it out!

By the way, if you have a passion for making products and want to consider selling them, please keep in mind that there are rules and regulations that must be followed. Testing for bacteria, product stability, and shelf life is necessary—as is including expiration dates on the labels. It is best to completely educate yourself on the law regarding safety of personal-care products.

FRESH-LEMON SURFACE STERILIZER

Makes 8 ounces

This simple recipe minimizes bacterial overgrowth in your homemade products.

> 1 cup Everclear alcohol, 190 proof (95% alcohol)
>
> 15 drops lemon essential oil
>
> 5 drops tea tree essential oil

Combine ingredients into a spray bottle, and shake well. Use this lemon spray to sterilize countertops, measuring utensils, pots, and anything else that needs a little extra cleansing. Spray all over the item or counter, and wipe off with a clean, dry cloth or paper towel.

When to Discard: in about a year

KITCHEN ITEMS YOU WILL NEED

Now that you know how to be mindful when making products, here are kitchen utensils and items you will need. When I was first starting out, I reused a lot of things I already had. I would clean out jars that I had in the kitchen or containers of products that had been used up. I labeled my products with Sharpie markers and utilized my canning jars. I did whatever I could to save money. I recommend doing the same if you are just starting out and do not want to spend a bunch of money on containers.

Canning jars are a great way to get started. I suggest getting the plastic, BPA-free freezer jar lids instead of using the metal canning lids. They definitely work better and can be reused by simply throwing them in the dishwasher. In the next section are a few things you may need when doing DIY recipes.

SUGGESTED ITEMS TO HAVE ON HAND

1 and 2 ounce glass dropper bottles

10 milliliter glass roller bottles

Bowls in various sizes

Cheesecloth and/or coffee filters

Eyedropper

Hand-held blender

Label maker

Mason jars in various sizes

Mason BPA-free plastic lids

Measuring spoons and cups

Notebooks

Pans that can get messy

Pretty wooden spoons/spatulas for removing product from jars

Sharpie markers

Silicone molds, large and small

Small and medium-sized funnels

Small glass and plastic containers

Spatulas for mixing

Spray/spritz bottles in various sizes

Stickers or labels

Whisks of various sizes

Wire-mesh handheld strainer

Below are some ingredients that I would recommend having on hand for DIY recipes. Many of these ingredients are listed in my favorite recipes provided in this book.

SUGGESTED INGREDIENTS TO HAVE ON HAND

Activated charcoal

Almond extract

Aloe vera

Apricot oil

Argan oil

Avocado oil

Bananas

Beetroot powder

Bentonite clay

Calendula oil/tincture

Castile soap

Cinnamon

Citric acid

Cocoa butter (wafers)

Coconut oil (raw, unrefined, and fractionated)

Colloidal silver

Diatomaceous earth

Epsom salts

Essential oils

Glycerin (food grade)

Grapeseed oil

Himalayan sea salt

Honey

Jojoba oil

Lavender flowers (dried)

Lemon juice

Magnesium chloride (magnesium flakes)

Nutmeg

Oats and oat flour

Olive oil

Orange extract

Peppermint leaves (dried)

Pumpkin

Rosehip seed oil

Rum

Sugar

Turmeric

Vanilla extract

Vitamin C powder

Vodka

Witch hazel

Xanthan gum

CHOOSING BETTER SKIN-CARE PRODUCTS AT THE STORE

Let's face it, most people cannot make every product they need—unless, of course, this is your passion, in which case I understand! Here are some tips for when you do buy commercially prepared skin-care products:

1. Find products that are aloe based or oil based vs. water-based. This means the first ingredient listed is an oil or aloe vera, not water. Ingredients are listed in order of the amount used in the products. So if aloe vera is the first item listed on the ingredient list, then that is the largest amount of ingredient used in the product. The last item listed would be the least amount of ingredient used.

2. If there are preservatives in the product, make sure they are toward the bottom of the list of ingredients. Look for products that do not include parabens or harsh chemicals.

3. Make sure most of the ingredients are "real," such as almond oil, coconut oil, aloe vera, pomegranate, or at least words you understand.

4. Be sure that the shelf life is not too far out. A product that will last five-plus years on a shelf is not something you want to put on your skin.

CHEMICALS

A GUIDE TO PERSONAL-CARE INGREDIENTS

There is quite a bit of controversy on the percentage of topical ingredients that are actually absorbed into the skin. In my research, I have seen everything from only 1 percent to 90 percent—literally! However, the bottom line is that if we are using products that contain chemicals, some of them *do* absorb into the skin. I think we can all agree: the fewer chemicals

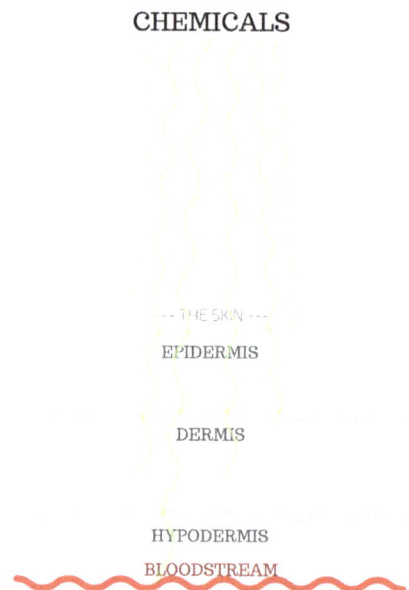

--- THE SKIN ---

EPIDERMIS

DERMIS

HYPODERMIS
BLOODSTREAM

How chemicals penetrate the skin and are absorbed into the bloodstream.

absorbed into the skin, the better. It is even more important that we are mindful of what we use on our children. A child's skin is more sensitive to what it absorbs. Not only that, but their young bodies are more sensitive as well. If children are absorbing chemicals from products, they may feel the effects more intensely than we adults do.

There are many harmful ingredients being included in everyday beauty products. As a concerned skin-care junkie, I want to share the ones I personally avoid at all times. Please note that manufacturers use a variety of different names to sneak these ingredients into our products. The Skin Deep website, created by the Environmental Working Group (www.EWG.org/skindeep) is a well-respected organization that provides good information about products and ingredients.

INGREDIENTS TO AVOID

Ingredient	Why I Avoid
Arsenic	Toxic to hormone balance and organs
Aluminum	Potentially toxic to the nervous system
Benzoyl peroxide	Can cause rash and irritation to the skin
Butylated hydroxyanisole (BHA), butylated hydroxytoluene (BHT)	Potentially toxic to hormone balance and organs
Para-aminobenzoic acid (PABA)	Carcinogenic
Parabens: methyl, butyl, ethyl, propyl	Potentially cancer causing and can interfere with hormones
Perfume and fragrance	Not closely regulated, but potentially toxic to organs and overall health
Petrochemicals: paraffin, mineral oil, petroleum, petrolatum, Vaseline	Potentially carcinogenic
Phthalates	Potentially cancer causing and can interfere with hormones
Propylene glycol (PG, PED, PPG) and butylene glycol (BG)	Irritants
Sodium laureth sulfate (SLS, SLES)	Irritant, potentially toxic to organs
Triclosan (aka "antibacterial")	Irritant, possibly toxic to hormone balance

My Number 1 Rule: Do Not Freak Out! I realize that many personal-care products contain these and other questionable ingredients. Switching out products is best taken in baby steps. What worked best for my family is what I like to call "replacement therapy," which is when you simply replace a completely used product with a healthier one each time you need a new one. Therefore, if you run out of facial cleanser, find a healthier, organic facial cleanser to replace it with or make your own. Use this same process with lotion, deodorant, serums, and so on.

The more clean and pure a product's ingredients are, the healthier and happier we will be. Take a look at the labels to see if a safer replacement product is necessary. See the glossary on page 210 for a complete index of ingredients.

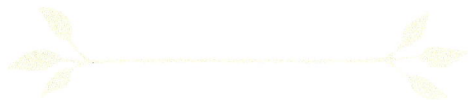

CHAPTER 3

All About Your Skin

The skin is our largest organ, and it protects us from the environment and outside elements. It regulates body temperature and allows us to recognize touch and to feel heat and cold. It is an amazing structure that shields our body. Our skin even protects us from bacteria and infection.

The skin has three layers; the epidermis, the dermis, and the hypodermis (subcutaneous fatty tissue).

The epidermis is the outermost layer of skin. It acts as the protective shield. The epidermis contains melanocytes, which are unique cells that produce our skin pigment. This pigment is called melanin. As a result, the epidermis is where you can see your unique skin tone and characteristics such as freckles.

The dermis is just beneath the epidermis. It contains connective tissue, lymph vessels, hair follicles, and sweat glands. The deeper layer is called the hypodermis or subcutaneous tissue. This deep layer is made up of collagen and fat tissue.

The layers of the skin are important to understand when you are taking care of yourself. It is good to know that the epidermis, or surface layer, of the skin

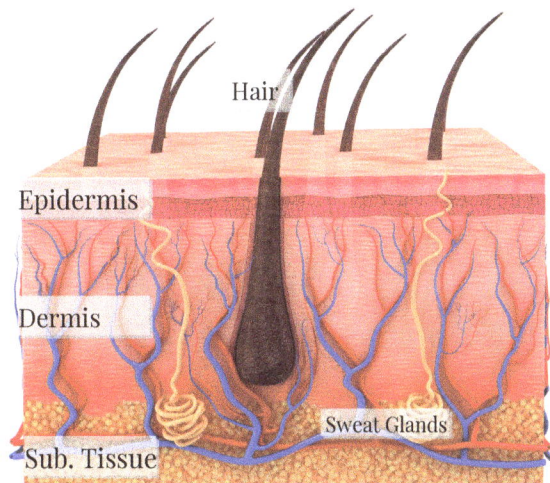

The layers of the skin

is the area you will be exfoliating and nourishing. You never want to go too deep into the epidermis and disrupt the deeper layers such as the dermis. Products that you put on the skin are absorbed through the top layer and penetrate into the deeper layers. Because of that, having a proper skin-care routine and healthy products is important for your skin's overall health.

COLLAGEN & PEPTIDES

Human skin is made up mostly of collagen, about 75 percent. Collagen is what gives our skin its thickness. It is a protein that is made of long segments of amino acids arranged like a chain. Collagen breaks down over time. The short segments of amino acids are the tiny proteins and active molecules known as peptides.

When collagen is depleted because of aging, environment, and excess exposure to the sun, it is not fully replaced. This causes the skin to thin and wrinkles to form. As collagen breaks down, it produces certain peptides. When we apply peptides topically to the skin, our body thinks we need to produce more collagen, sort of like a red-flag indicator to repair the skin. In a way, you are tricking the skin into a more youthful appearance. For this reason, many skin-care companies are offering products containing peptides.

Peptides are extremely hydrophilic, which means water soluble. Because they are very small in size, peptides can penetrate the skin's protective barriers to get to the deeper layers of the dermis. Peptides are sensitive to heat and can easily break down, so in order to be functional, they must be stabilized. As a result, most peptides that are used in skin-care products are naturally derived but are for the most part synthetic. Two commonly used peptides in skin care are palmitoyl pentapeptide and palmitoyl oligopeptide. Both peptides are intended to reduce fine lines and wrinkles.

Vitamin C also plays a big role in building amino acids, and deficiency of vitamin C interferes with collagen production. Research shows that there are many foods you can eat to boost collagen production, including citrus foods that contain vitamin C. Here are a few more foods to consider if you want to naturally replenish collagen, from the inside out, by eating nutritious food.

• Berries	• Garlic
• Bone broth	• Organic Greek yogurt
• Chlorella (green algae)	• Organic milk
• Citrus fruits	• Salmon
• Eggs	• Spinach and kale

Research is unclear on whether you can use actual food topically (instead of lab-generated peptides) to trick the skin into producing more collagen. However, milk and similar foods, such as yogurt, contain important proteins and properties that can be similar to man-made peptides. For that reason, many of my recipes call for milk or yogurt. It is undeniable that a healthy diet can be the most beneficial in keeping collagen production at a healthy rate. Try some of the delicious smoothie recipes in chapter 18, which help to assist collagen production from the inside, while you target the outside with my recipes for collagen-enhancing creams for the neck and eyes.

SKIN CARE IN FRANCE

French women are known for having beautiful skin, and for good reason. They are taught to take good care of their skin at an early age. That usually does *not* include complicated skin-care routines or products full of unnecessary ingredients. In fact, French women love simplicity and pure ingredients. They take their skin-care products, routines, and facial services very seriously. Additionally, they prefer facials over harsh treatments such as Botox, laser treatments, or chemical peels. Isabelle Bellis, a French celebrity epidemiologist and owner of the Isabelle Bellis Center in New York, says, "French women are obsessed with face massage to maintain a healthy glow and skin-tissue health and to relieve facial stress."

Reading about French (and European) skin care always warms my heart because these beautiful ladies are also in love with skin care and prefer facials over most popular spa services. Mireille Guiliano, author of *French Women Don't Get Facelifts*, states, "I'd rather have one facial a year than six manicures because it's almost like, if you take the analogy with the car, a yearly tune-up and you need it. It's not an indulgence. The basic ritual in a French home is to clean your skin every night."

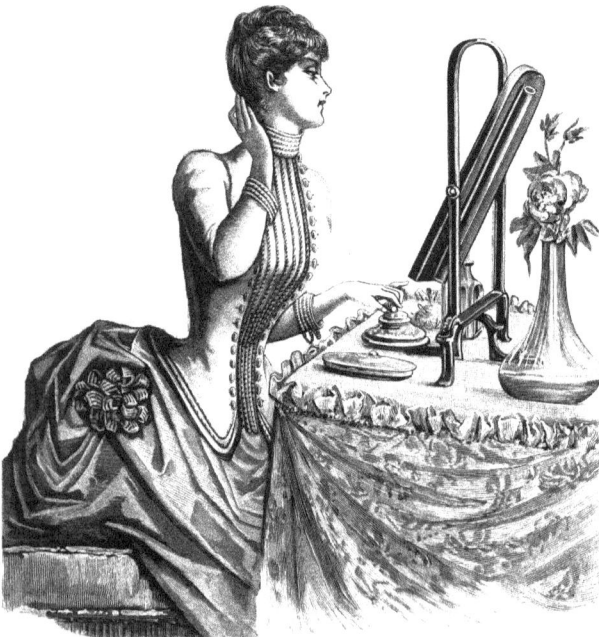

Guiliano believes in keeping it simple, and I completely agree. Pure ingredients are best when it comes to skin care. If there were two things I could recommend to my clients, it would be to always wash your face at night and always put on a good serum before getting your beauty sleep, especially if you have dry or mature skin. One of my personal beauty secrets is applying a blend of pure oils every night before bed. That is why you will find many suggested oil serums in this book.

CHAPTER 4

ROUTINE FOR YOUR SKIN TYPE

A s a professional esthetician, I have noticed patterns, trends, and misconceptions about caring for and maintaining healthy skin. The most common questions I get are "What is a skin-care routine?" and "What are the best products for me?"

Additionally, clients are curious about the products themselves and what they are intended to do. Throughout this book, I will go over each type of product and its use. Let us first dive into the different skin-care routines and which one is right for you. There are many different regimens for skin care, but I will discuss the two most common which work for either men or women.

The word *regimen* is from the Latin *regere*, which means "to rule." According to the dictionary, *regimen* means a plan or set of rules about food, exercise, or health to make someone become or stay at their optimum health.

I do not believe we need to be so extreme as to call a skin-care routine a *rule*. Instead, think of it as a healthy habit. In my opinion, there are two basic types of skin-care regimens: *maintenance* or *treatment*. Take the following simple test to determine if you want to maintain or treat your skin.

MAINTAIN OR TREAT QUESTIONNAIRE

1. Age Range

A. 28 years old or younger

B. Between 29–39 years old

C. 40 years or older

2. Skin Type (Unsure? Turn to page 33 to determine your skin type.)

A. Normal

B. Oily or combination

C. Dry

3. Skin Issues

A. No trouble areas

B. Fine lines, large pores, dull skin

C. Acne, rosacea, discoloration, sun damage

4. Diet

A. Mostly fruits, vegetables, lean meats

B. Balanced meals, some sugar and fast foods

C. Mostly fast food and/or processed foods

5. Lifestyle

A. Mostly a relaxed, steady-paced lifestyle

B. Somewhat hectic, balanced lifestyle

C. Busy, fast-paced, somewhat stressful lifestyle

6. Skin Elasticity

A. Overall skin tightness is in great shape

B. Under eyes, jawline, and neck area are a bit loose; fine lines

C. Sagging skin and deeper lines

7. Texture

A. My skin generally feels smooth

B. My skin generally feels smooth, but I have a few rough patches

C. My skin generally feels rough and bumpy all over

If the majority of your answers are A, you will want to *maintain* your skin. If the majority of your answers are B, you will want to consider *treating* your skin or using a few treatment options in your routine. If the majority of your answers are C, it is best to have a *treatment* plan in place. When in doubt, the ultimate question is: Do you want to see changes or improvement in your skin?

Most of us want to see improvement and generally go with the more involved skin-care regimen. However, when you are young or if you do not have time for a more involved routine and have always taken good care of your skin, a maintenance routine will work perfectly. Maintenance is generally to uphold the skin's current state and slow down aging, breakouts, discoloration, or sagging.

Maintenance Regimen

Step 1: Cleanse

Step 2: Moisturize

Step 3: Eye Treatment (optional)

This routine will keep your skin looking nice and will generally keep you free of breakouts and discoloration. However, if you have troubled skin, you will most likely need a treatment regimen to help balance your skin. For a treatment regimen, simply include the serums, scrubs and masks.

Treatment Regimen

Step 1: Cleanse

Step 2: Mask or Scrub

Step 3: Tone

Step 4: Serum

Step 5: Moisturize

Step 6: Eye Treatment

Regular facials or skin treatments from a licensed professional also help tremendously for either regimen. Facial massage and extractions can be very beneficial for the skin. As you can see from the two different routines, there is a small difference when you want better results.

NIGHTTIME VS. MORNING ROUTINE

One important thing to understand is that your nighttime routine is *way* more important than your morning routine. Your skin cells are regenerating while you sleep, so make sure you have on a wonderful serum and night cream before you go to bed and let your body do the rest of the work. There really is such a thing as "beauty sleep." So get your butt off the couch and go wash your face before you go to bed because it will make all the difference!

Choose the routine/regimen that works best for you—one that you will stick to regularly. Consistency is important with skin care. If you forget to wash your face a couple of days a week, you will see negative results.

How Much Product

Many clients ask how much product to use when doing a skin care routine. I am a little generous with these amounts, and you can definitely get away with less product if you choose. This is just a simple guide that I have found useful. These amounts should cover the entire face and *décolletage*, a French word that refers to the area that includes the neck, shoulders, upper back, and upper chest.

Product	How Much to Use
Cleanser	Almond size
Mask & scrub	Walnut size
Toner	Couple of spritzes on face or on cotton ball
Serum	Pea size
Moisturizer	Blueberry size
Eye cream	Sunflower-seed size
Sunscreen	Blueberry size (for face)

WHAT'S YOUR SKIN TYPE?

Knowing your skin type before you choose the products you want to use will help you get the best results. Skin type can also be affected by the climate you live in. For example, many of my clients in Colorado suffer from dry skin. Our environment is pretty dry compared to many other places, and we have frequent high winds that do not help matters. Those who live in climates with more humidity, such as near the coastal areas, may have more trouble with oily skin. Even though climate plays a role in our skin-care routines, it does not always determine our skin type.

Skin Type	How It Feels	Helpful Products	Helpful Ingredients
Oily	Your skin feels oily most of the time. You are consistently fighting shine or greasiness. You feel that your face needs frequent washing.	A gentle cleanser, a salt or sugar scrub, gentle enzyme masks, a rotating brush for cleansing, light serums, moisturizers	Frankincense, aloe vera, lavender, tea tree, lemon, grapeseed oil, peppermint
Dry	Your skin is dry with flaky patches. Skin regularly feels tight or itchy. More fine lines around eye and mouth area.	A moisturizing cleanser, a sugar scrub, a rotating brush for cleansing, moisturizing masks, oil serums, heavier night creams	Honey, jojoba oil, almond oil, lavender, chamomile, banana, oats
Normal	No real trouble with oil or dryness, easy to take care of skin without regular breakouts.	A gentle cleanser, sugar scrubs, enzyme masks, light serums, nighttime moisturizer	Most ingredients will be good to use on normal skin.

Skin Type	How It Feels	Helpful Products	Helpful Ingredients
Combination	Part of the face is dry or normal, and part is oily. It's a constant battle trying to balance the skin.	Salt or sugar scrubs, gentle enzyme masks, a rotating brush for cleansing, light serums, oil serums, night-time moisturizers	Aloe vera, calendula, witch hazel, chamomile, lavender, jojoba oil
Sensitive	Any of the above skin types can have sensitive skin. Sensitive skin becomes red easily if touched. It also can be easily injured and bleed more readily. Those with sensitive skin tend to "blush" more often and burn easily in the sun.	A moisturizing cleanser, a rotating brush for cleansing (used lightly), calming oils and serums, heavy night cream.	Calendula, oats, chamomile, carrot seed oil, honey, banana and jojoba oil

Knowing your skin type can help enhance your results. If you are using a harsh cleanser and have sensitive skin, that may be causing a breakout or dryness.

THE HEALING ART OF FACIAL MASSAGE

Another thing to consider in your routine is getting regular massages, whether it's a full-body massage or just a facial. There are surprisingly more benefits to massage than you may think. Most of us love the relaxing atmosphere and leave the spa with a glowing complexion. Facials and massages can help relieve stress and keep the skin youthful. Additionally, they help relieve muscle tension, increase circulation, offer headache relief, and help detoxify the body.

Massage lifts the spirit. Calming music, aromatherapy, and touch have a way of healing a person from the outside in. Many of us have a hard time taking a time-out from work, family, social media, and the stress of life. Having a spa treatment forces us to shut off everything and enjoy that moment.

Just like the body, the face can use a little love from time to time. Massage movement can increase blood flow and circulation to the face and warm up the color of the skin. Facial treatments will slough off dead skin cells and help with fine lines and wrinkles, giving the complexion a more youthful appearance. It also stimulates the muscles and sinuses, which can help relieve congestion and allergies.

Massaging the temples and tight muscles on the face, shoulders, and neck can help relieve headaches and may help relieve TMJ (temporomandibular joints), which can be caused from jaw clenching or talking for extended periods of time. Regular massage to relax the muscles is extremely beneficial. Another great benefit is the stimulation of the lymph system.

The Lymph System

The lymphatic system is a large network of vessels and nodes throughout the body. This complex system is directly linked to your immune system. The lymphatic system allows your body to detoxify by helping to remove waste buildup from body tissue. This is all dependent on other body systems such as blood pressure within the cardiovascular system and how well the overall circulatory system is working. If your other systems are not functioning well it can lead to a slower lymph system that has a delayed detoxification process.

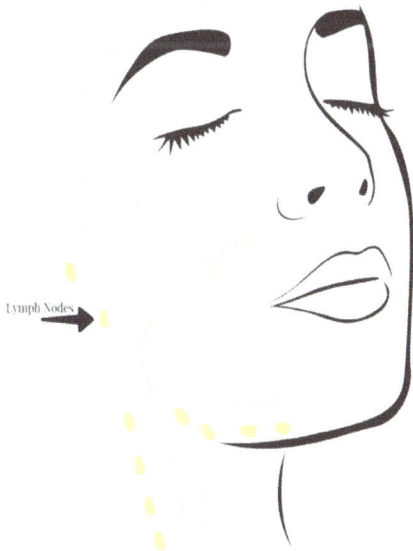

This is where manual stimulation of the lymph nodes can be extremely helpful. Gentle massage can help speed up the process of the lymph system by eliminating toxins from the body. Your immune system is boosted and inflammation in that area is reduced. When the lymph system is slow, fluid accumulates in the tissue and can result in swelling in the affected area. When fluid builds up, it can cause discomfort, irritation, puffiness, and a dull complexion.

Lymph Nodes

Direction for lymph massage drainage

A lymph-friendly facial should offer a gentle, soothing, relaxing massage, which can reduce swelling in the eye and neck area, as well as in the rest of the face. Having a boosted immune system is an extra bonus. There are other ways to stimulate the lymph system, such as dry brushing.

Some people prefer dry brushing as a way to stimulate the lymphatic system because it is simple and quick enough to be done on a daily basis. Dry brushing is where you brush dry, bare skin with a soft-bristled handheld brush. Personally I do not prefer this method. In my opinion, massage is much more enjoyable and relaxing.

In general, gentle lymphatic drainage should consist of movements that move toward the heart. Pressure should be gentle yet firm. Lymph drainage should not hurt or be uncomfortable. When focusing on the face, movements should be directional to the outside edge of the face where most lymph nodes are located; then it should move down the neck and away from the face.

GIVE YOURSELF A LYMPH-DRAINING FACIAL

Clean your face with a gentle cleanser. Apply an oil serum, such as the Glowing-Skin Oil Serum on page 82.

Begin at the top center area of the forehead. With medium-gentle pressure, bring your first three fingers of each hand across the eyebrow ridge repeatedly for fifteen seconds.

Follow with medium-gentle pressure from your ring fingers underneath the eye area, right above the cheekbones repeatedly for fifteen seconds.

Using your ring and middle finger, begin in the center of your eyebrows and gently slide fingers toward the outside edge of the face, tracing above your eyebrows to the temple area. Repeat five to ten times.

With your first three fingers, make long, downward strokes from right underneath your cheekbones toward the neck area. Repeat five to ten times.

With your first two fingers, apply medium to light pressure to the outside of the jaw area. Make a few circular movements and then move down toward the neck. Repeat five to ten times.

Repeat the massage, if desired. Drink plenty of water after you do the lymph-drainage facial to assist in removing waste, toxins, and excess water from the body.

KEEP YOUR NECK YOUTHFUL

One of the most obvious signs of aging is when the skin on our neck begins to wrinkle. As we age, skin elasticity weakens, making the neck area appear loose and weathered. Aging is often most noticeable on the face, neck, and décolletage. Surprisingly, the skin on our neck is different from our face as there are fewer sebaceous glands, which produce the oil that naturally lubricates the skin. Lack of oil can cause the skin to age more quickly, causing the neck to need special treatment.

Thankfully there are a few things you can do to keep your neck and chest area looking youthful. First, always include this area in your daily skin-care routine. Second, exfoliate. The neck can be more vulnerable to dryness and dead skin cell accumulation. Exfoliating often will help rejuvenate and smooth the skin.

Vitamins C and E are also helpful for the neck area. Applying important vitamins to the skin will help stimulate collagen reproduction, which will increase firmness. Having products that contain these essential vitamins can help keep the neck looking young. Diet also plays a big role in overall skin health. Eating foods high in vitamin A and beta-carotene, including fruits and vegetables such as berries and carrots, may increase cell turnover. Additionally, consuming an antioxidant-packed diet will help protect your skin. Foods high in essential fatty acids (alpha-linolenic and linoleic fatty acids), such as walnuts or olive oil, will also help skin cells stay hydrated and glowing. Consuming enough water every day will help as well.

As previously mentioned, facial exercises and massage are beneficial. Getting regular facials is useful for cell turnover and increased blood flow. Additionally, regular exercise ultimately firms your neck when you are working out your whole body. Doing something physically active every day helps the skin stay youthful.

Keeping your head up throughout the day is also important. We are constantly looking down at phones, laptops, or even books. This can be hard on your neck as well as your spine. Horizontal wrinkles can develop on your neck from inactivity because the neck's skin and muscles are thinner than the skin on your face.

Last but not least, avoid wool and rough fabrics that can irritate the neck area. When the neck gets irritated we are more likely to pull at the skin or damage it. Wear loose cotton or breathable fabrics around the neck and décolletage. For a wonderful neck treatment, try the Nighty-Night Neck Mask on page 102.

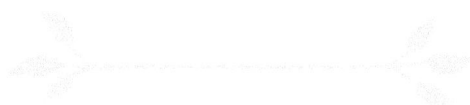

CHAPTER 5

YOUR SKIN

Cleansing is the first step in the facial routine. Removing accumulated daily dirt, oil, and pollution from your face and décolletage can be beneficial. Unfortunately, finding a decent cleanser can be a difficult task. Most of us have come to love the thick, pretty-smelling, foaming cleansers that leave the face feeling squeaky clean. We have been taught to cleanse with a strong cleanser so that we do not get breakouts. Sadly, this is a misconception.

That squeaky-clean feeling can be drying. When the skin dries out, oil production increases and can cause an imbalance, which can cause breakouts. In addition to finding a gentle cleanser that will not dry out your skin, it is important to have a product that is not full of chemicals. The ingredients some companies use in cleansers can be pretty harmful. In order to get that scented, thick, beautiful lather, they have to put in a lot of not-so-pretty ingredients.

AN ESTHETICIAN'S OPINION ON INGREDIENTS

When I first see clients for a facial, I always ask what skin-care products they are using, especially if they are having trouble with their skin. Many of them buy typical products sold at supermarkets that are easily accessible and reasonably priced. Before I became an esthetician obsessed with natural ingredients, I also bought these products, especially if they were on sale.

Typical cleansers often are water based and contain a plethora of lab-made ingredients such as sodium sulfonate, phosphate, propylene glycol, parabens, artificial color, and fragrance. The hidden chemicals in store-bought cleansers are just another great reason to make your own. Cleansers do not need to be complicated; in fact, you may love a cleanser with just one or two ingredients, such as an oil cleanser. Oil cleansing usually requires only one or two rich oils. Give the following all-natural cleanser recipes a try and pick your favorite.

LAVENDER FACIAL WIPES

Makes about 20 wipes

A friend of mine asked me if I had a handy recipe for safer, more natural face wipes to use when she is at the gym and needs to quickly remove makeup. I created this one because it removes makeup and moisturizes at the same time. That way the only product you need are the face wipes and maybe a moisturizer if you have dry skin. Packing a cleanser, serum, moisturizer, and toner is inconvenient for most people on the go.

½ cup pure aloe juice

½ cup distilled water

½ tablespoon castile soap (lavender or unscented)

1 teaspoon apricot oil

1 teaspoon witch hazel

5–7 drops lavender essential oil

1 box of thick, absorbent Kleenex Hand Towels or dry baby wipes

Combine all ingredients, except towels, in a bowl.

Fold 10 Kleenex Hand Towels or dry baby wipes and soak in the liquid mixture until towels are completely drenched. Wring out excess liquid but leave the towels very damp so they do not dry out too quickly. Store in a resealable Ziplock bag and carry them in your gym bag, in your car, or by your bedside for late nights when you do not feel like washing your face.

To use these as sanitizer wipes for hands, add tea tree essential oil which can act as an antimicrobial.

When to Discard: about 1 week

THE BENEFITS OF OIL CLEANSING

Oil cleansing may go against everything you have ever learned. At least it did for me. Growing up, I learned that oil-free products were better because they did not make you break out and that your cleanser should always be super-soapy. However, this is actually not true. Research continues to uncover the amazing benefits of oil on the skin.

Oil cleansing is very simple. You need only a warm, damp washcloth and an oil that works well with your skin. Putting oil on your skin will actually lift excess oil, makeup, dead skin, and pollutants. A recommended oil blend to use is a combination of olive oil and castor oil. Olive oil is great for cleansing, while castor oil is great at protecting and moisturizing the skin. Another popular option is to pair almond oil and jojoba oil.

HYDRATING OLIVE OIL CLEANSER

Makes enough for one use

½ teaspoon olive oil

½ teaspoon castor oil

Combine ingredients and liberally distribute over your entire face and décolletage. Massage until the oil is well absorbed into the skin. Use a warm, damp washcloth to wipe away excess oil. Pat dry, and apply serum and moisturizer if needed.

You can make this recipe in a larger batch and keep it in your bathroom for easy access.

When to Discard: about 6–12 months, depending on the shelf life of your oils

GLOWING-REPAIR OIL CLEANSER

Makes 4 ounces

¼ cup olive oil

¼ cup castor oil

1 tablespoon carrot seed oil

5 drops lemon essential oil

5 drops rosemary essential oil

Combine all ingredients, and store in a reusable container with a lid. Liberally distribute about 1 to 2 teaspoons over your entire face area, including décolletage. Massage until well absorbed into the skin. Use a warm, damp washcloth to wipe away excess oil. Pat dry, and apply serum and moisturizer if needed.

When to Discard: about 6–12 months (depending on the shelf life of your oils)

FACIAL CLEANSERS

Cleansing can be a fun part of your skin-care routine. If you are not a fan of oil cleansing, give a few of these alternative recipes a try. Using circular, gentle motions while cleansing will help to slough off dead skin cells, open up the pores and rejuvenate the skin. Take your time while cleansing and remember to pamper yourself.

SWEET & GENTLE FACIAL CLEANSER

Makes 2 ounces

¼ cup almond oil

1 tablespoon castile soap
(lavender or unscented)

1½ tablespoons raw honey

6 drops lavender or vanilla
essential oil

Combine all ingredients, and save the mixture in a container with a lid. Use as a normal cleanser with your facial routine.

You can easily turn this recipe into a citrus facial cleanser by replacing the lavender castile soap with citrus castile soap and using 6 drops of wild orange essential oil, instead of using lavender or vanilla essential oil.

When to Discard: about 2 weeks

HONEY-COCONUT FACIAL SCRUB

Makes enough for one use

1 tablespoon raw, unrefined
organic coconut oil

½ teaspoon baking soda

½ tablespoon raw honey

½ tablespoon unscented castile soap

3 drops benzoin essential oil (optional)

Combine all ingredients. Gently massage facial scrub onto skin in circular motions. Rinse thoroughly. Use this scrub as a normal cleanser with your daily facial routine or as a treatment scrub one to two times per week.

When to Discard: about 5 days

GENTLE ACNE FACIAL CLEANSER

Makes 6 ounces

¼ cup aloe vera gel

½ tablespoon glycerin

1 tablespoon olive oil

1 teaspoon baking soda

¼ cup castile soap
(unscented or almond)

10 drops tea tree essential oil

Combine all ingredients and mix well. Store in a container with a lid, but do not put the lid on it for about an hour to allow the baking soda to settle.

Use as a normal cleanser with your facial routine. Shake the container gently before each use.

When to Discard: about 2 weeks

SWEET ALMOND EXFOLIATING MILK

Makes 6 ounces

1/4 cup raw unrefined
coconut oil

1/4 cup almond castile soap

1 tablespoon sweetened
condensed milk

1 tablespoon aloe vera gel

1 teaspoon baking soda

1/2 teaspoon almond extract

Heat coconut oil in a saucepan on low, just until the oil is melted. Remove from heat and add remaining ingredients. Stir all ingredients thoroughly. Transfer to a container with a lid, but do not put the lid on it for about an hour to allow the baking soda to settle and the mixture to completely cool.

Use as a normal cleanser with your facial routine. Shake container gently before each use.

When to Discard: about 2 weeks

CHAPTER 6

Using Toner in Your

SKIN-CARE ROUTINE

The main purpose of toner, which is applied after cleansing, is to balance the skin—in other words, to keep it clear of pimples and looking healthy. Think of toner as a way of deepening the cleansing step. Use a toner when your skin feels extra greasy or you are trying to clear up a breakout of pimples.

Do you *have* to use a toner? No, you do not. And you do not have to use toner all the time. You can simply use it when you feel your skin needs a little extra love. Some people like to include this step in their everyday skincare routine because it helps their skin stay balanced.

There are so many toner options on the market that it can be pretty overwhelming to figure out which one to get, if any at all. Toner usually has a water-like consistency and is either sprayed on the face or rubbed on with a cotton ball or facial pads. It is generally not rinsed off.

Choose a toner that has pure ingredients such as witch hazel or apple cider vinegar. Many companies sell witch hazel with added fillers and chemicals. Make sure when you buy your witch hazel that it is labeled "100 percent pure." Witch hazel is a great go-to toner because it is gentle enough for all skin types but effective enough for even super-oily skin.

If you need something a little stronger and are fighting sun or age spots, try my Simple Brightening Lemon Toner on page 47. Also, it is important to note that some toners can cause your skin to be sensitive to the sun. For that reason, make sure you wear your SPF sunblock during the day and/or use the toner only in the evening for extra caution.

TONER BENEFITS

- Shrinks pores
- Balances skin pH
- Provides a blast of vitamins
- Removes excess dirt and oil
- Refreshes skin
- Helps skin absorb products
- Helps minimize ingrown hairs
- Clears up breakouts
- Removes dead skin cells
- Adds moisture

Using a toner can help the absorption of other products such as serums and moisturizers. Using a gentle cleanser or wiping your face with a warm washcloth can also help with absorption. In my opinion, however, using a toner goes a tiny step further in preparing your skin for the products.

Many people think of toners as harsh products that smell like alcohol and give you a tight face. If this is happening to you after you use a toner, it is all wrong for you. A toner should not cause irritation or dry out your face. A toner should not burn your eyes or reek of alcohol.

DANGERS OF USING THE WRONG TONER

- Skin irritation
- Redness
- Breakouts
- Eye irritation
- Dry skin
- Imbalanced skin

If you experience any of these issues after using a toner, stop using it immediately and allow your skin to heal. Try a mild toner such as pure witch hazel (as discussed above) or one of the DIY recipes. Overall, I think having a toner in your regular skin-care routine is extremely beneficial, especially if you struggle with combination or oily skin.

SIMPLE BRIGHTENING LEMON TONER

Makes 8 ounces

½ cup 100 percent pure witch hazel

½ cup pure organic lemon juice

Combine ingredients in a container with a flip-top lid. Shake lightly before each use.

After cleansing, apply toner solution to a cotton ball and apply to face and décolletage.

When to Discard: about 3 months

CITRUS FACIAL TONER

The Citrus Facial Toner is a fresh-smelling toner that helps to brighten and nourish the skin.

Makes 4 ounces

¼ cup aloe juice	½ teaspoon vitamin E
¼ cup lemon juice	½ teaspoon rosehip seed oil
½ teaspoon carrot seed oil	1 ½ teaspoons 80-proof vodka
½ teaspoon colloidal silver	10 drops orange essential oil

Combine all ingredients. Put in a container with a sealable lid and give it a little shake. After cleansing, apply toner solution to a cotton ball and apply to face and décolletage with your evening routine. Shake before each use.

When to Discard: about 2 months

ACNE-CLEARING VANILLA TONER

Makes 5 ounces

> 1 tablespoon colloidal silver
>
> ½ cup witch hazel
>
> 1 teaspoon vanilla extract
>
> ¼ dropper infused white willow bark tincture (½ teaspoon)*
>
> 7 drops vanilla essential oil (optional)

Combine all ingredients and pour into a dark container with a sealable lid. (Keeping colloidal silver in a dark container helps preserve its shelf life.)

After cleansing, apply toner solution to a cotton ball (or spritz directly on troubled areas) and apply to face and décolletage. Shake before each use.

*To make your own infused White Willow Bark Tincture see page 158.

When to Discard: about 3 months

SOOTHING FENNEL BALANCING TONER

Makes 8 ounces

> ½ cup aloe vera juice
>
> ¼ cup fennel tincture (see page 160)
>
> 5 drops rosemary essential oil
>
> 3 drops sage essential oil

Combine all ingredients. Put in a container with a sealable lid.

After cleansing, apply toner solution to a cotton ball—or spritz directly on troubled areas—and apply to face and décolletage. Shake before each use.

When to Discard: about 3 months

SOOTHING ROSE FACIAL SPRITZER

Makes 8 ounces

1 cup rose hydrosol (see page 153)

10 drops rose essential oil*

10 drops lavender essential oil

Combine all ingredients and pour into a spritz bottle. Spray face and décolletage morning and evening, or whenever needed.

Most rose essential oil is blended with another oil. Pure rose essential oil is extremely expensive and you would only need one or two drops versus ten of the blended.

When to Discard: about 6 months

PAMPER YOUR SKIN WITH A FACIAL STEAM

Another great way to balance the skin is with an herbal facial steam, which can help restore moisture, promote repair of damaged skin, and bring oxygen to the skin, giving an overall younger appearance.

Generally my clients enjoy a facial steam for five to ten minutes in the spa. If you happen to have a tabletop steamer, it's much more convenient than heating water in a small pot and putting your face near it with a towel over your head. However, heating your own water in a pot makes it easy for you to add as many skin enhancing herbs as desired. Commonly used botanicals for a facial steam include lavender, chamomile, fennel, peppermint, thyme, rosemary and rose petals.

The only danger of doing a facial steam is heating up the skin too much or too often, especially if you suffer from severe acne or rosacea. Those with sensitive skin should also use caution and steam for only about five minutes at a time. Use organically grown herbs in your steam because you are breathing these in as well as absorbing steam into the skin. Typically, dried herbs are used in a facial steam because they are more convenient. You can use fresh herbs as well, although you will want to double the amount used.

If you double your dried-herb batch, it is easy to keep extra on hand for the next time you steam your face. For a unique gift, place dried herbs in a pretty package, along with my instructions.

SKIN-CALMING FACIAL STEAM

Makes enough for one use

> 2 teaspoons dried organic lavender flowers
>
> 1 large sprig organic fresh rosemary, or
> 1 teaspoon dried organic rosemary
>
> 2–4 organic rosebud heads, fresh or dried

Cleanse your face. Place 3 cups of water in a pot, and bring to a boil. Let the water boil for a minute to purify it before stirring in the herbs. Allow them to simmer on low for a minute before removing from heat.

Place the hot herbal pot in a stable place where you are able to sit comfortably for several minutes. Drape a large tea towel over your head to create a sort of tent. Place face about 12 inches from the edge of the pot to allow steam to envelop the skin, while relaxing with your eyes closed. Gently dab excess water from your face and proceed with serum and moisturizer and/or your everyday skin-care routine.

When to Discard: Dried herbs will keep for several years. Add them to water when you're ready to do a facial steam.

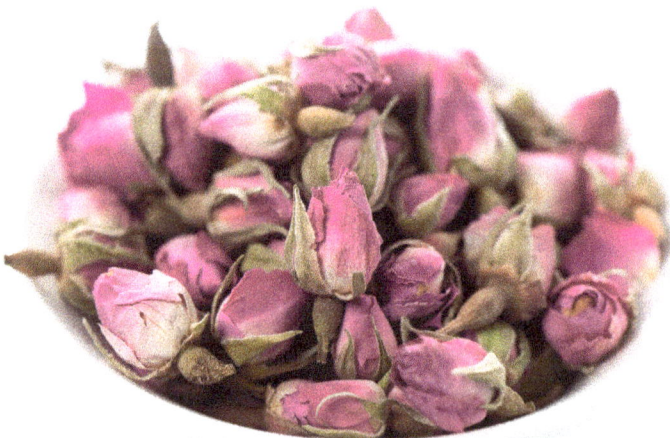

YOUNG & REFRESHED FACIAL STEAM

Makes enough for one use

> 2 teaspoons dried fennel seeds
>
> 1 teaspoon crushed dried peppermint leaves
>
> 1 teaspoon whole cloves

Cleanse your face. Place 3 cups of water in a pot, and bring to a boil. Let the water boil for a minute to purify it before stirring in the herbs. Allow them to steep in the water for a minute before removing from heat.

Place the hot herbal pot in a stable place where you are able to sit comfortably for several minutes. Drape a large tea towel over your head to create a sort of tent. Place your face about 12 inches from the edge of the pot to allow steam to envelop the skin, while relaxing with your eyes closed. Gently dab excess water from your face and proceed with serum and moisturizer and/or your everyday skin-care routine.

When to Discard: Dried herbs will keep for several years. Add them to water when you're ready to do a facial steam.

CRISP HERBAL FACIAL STEAM

Makes enough for one use

1 teaspoon dried organic chamomile

1 teaspoon dried organic peppermint leaves

1 teaspoon dried organic lavender flowers

½ teaspoon dried organic nettle

Cleanse your face. Place 3 cups of water in a pot, and bring to a boil. Let the water boil for a minute to purify it before stirring in the herbs. Allow them to steep in the water for a minute before removing from heat.

Place the hot herbal pot in a stable place where you are able to sit comfortably for several minutes. Drape a large tea towel over your head to create a sort of tent. Place your face about 12 inches from the edge of the pot to allow steam to envelop the skin, while relaxing with your eyes closed. Gently dab excess water from your face and proceed with serum and moisturizer and/or your everyday skin-care routine.

When to Discard: Dried herbs will keep for several years. Add them to water when you're ready to do a facial steam.

CHAPTER 7

Exfoliating Your Skin

Exfoliating is one of the easiest things you can do to instantly improve the texture and appearance of your skin. There are many benefits to exfoliating. However, it is important to note some of the dangers as well. Extreme exfoliating has become quite popular. Microdermabrasion, harsh chemical peels, derma-planing, and laser treatments are the procedures that bring in the most money for a licensed professional in the skin-care world. Unfortunately, some of these procedures may not be the best option for the client. When exfoliation is done gently and correctly, it can be one of the best things you do for your complexion. When done incorrectly or for too long a period, it can cause serious harm.

BENEFITS TO EXFOLIATION

• Removes dead skin cells

• Helps keep the pores clear, which helps with acne and breakouts

• Increases circulation

• Stimulates cell turnover

• Helps even out skin tone and discoloration

• Gives the skin a beautiful glow

• Keeps the skin soft and supple

• Helps minimize fine lines and wrinkles

Many times when trying to reverse skin damage from sun, scarring, or discoloration, we think we need extreme measures to see results. But this is not necessarily true. It is important to remember that it took time to create damage to the skin—and it will take time to reverse it.

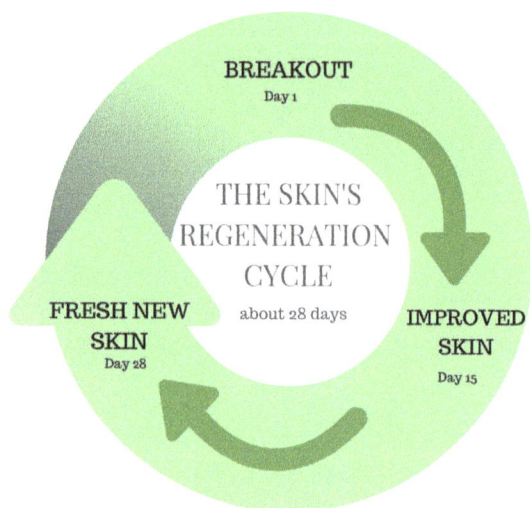

THE SKIN'S
REGENERATION
CYCLE
about 28 days

BREAKOUT
Day 1

IMPROVED
SKIN
Day 15

FRESH NEW
SKIN
Day 28

The skin's regeneration cycle

The cell-regeneration cycle of the skin takes about 28 days for middle-aged adults. You will see immediate results from exfoliation, but it may take about a month to see the full results.

This illustration shows the regeneration cycle for the skin of an average adult. Younger skin regenerates more quickly. For example a teenager's skin may go through the regeneration cycle every fifteen days, while a mature adult in their sixties may take up to sixty-five days to regenerate the surface of their skin.

The outer layer of the epidermis is made up of dead skin cells that flake or wash off. The new cells in the lower portion of the epidermis move upward to the outside of the skin. These fresh, new cells give the skin a softer, more youthful appearance. That's why exfoliating your skin can help dead skin cells fall off earlier, encouraging the new cells to move to the surface.

DANGERS OF OVER-EXFOLIATION

- Inflammation

- Scarring

- Redness

- Burning

- Unnecessary peeling

- Sensitivity

- Painful skin lacerations

Getting to know your skin's sensitivity level and knowing your skin type can help tremendously. Do *not* expect every skin-care professional to know your skin the minute they look at it. Fighting for the best care for your skin type is key to getting the best results when seeing a professional.

TWO TYPES OF EXFOLIANTS

1. Chemical Exfoliants. Chemical exfoliants dissolve keratin protein and break up dead skin cells a little differently than the physical (mechanical) exfoliants. Chemical exfoliants usually contain ingredients such as alpha hydroxy acids (AHAs) and beta hydroxy acids (BHAs). Sometimes these chemical exfoliants are synthetic, though some are derived from natural sources, as is the case with enzyme masks that contain pineapple, papaya, or pumpkin.

Chemical Exfoliants	
AHAs	Naturally occurring acids derived from fruits, milk and sugarcane (glycolic acid, lactic acid, tartaric acid, citric acid, malic acid, and mandelic acid). AHAs are water soluble.
BHAs	BHAs go a little deeper into the pores to remove dead skin cells and excess sebum (salicylic and citric). BHAs are oil soluble.
Stronger chemical acids	There are a variety of acids that can be used. Not all are safe, in my opinion. These can include resorcinol, pyruvic acid, trichloroacetic acid, or carbolic acid (phenol).
Enzymes	Enzymes act as "biological catalysts," which means that it speeds up the skin's natural repair and helps to naturally exfoliate in the process. Popular enzymes are pineapple, papaya, and pumpkin.

2. Mechanical Exfoliants. Usually referred to as scrubs, these products include ingredients such as salt, sugar, finely ground grains, beads, and even fine sand.

Mechanical Exfoliants	
Microdermabrasion	Microderm is performed with an expensive machine, generally either the crystal microdermabrasion technology or a diamond-tip microdermabrasion. This procedure should always be done under the care of a licensed professional, ideally someone who has had extensive training on the machine they use and who know how it performs on clients with various skin types.
Brushes or gloves	A rotating brush can be a great option because you can move it very lightly over the skin. Because of the rapid movement, a rotating brush can clean pores and stimulate blood flow. Exfoliating gloves can vary, so be careful not to get gloves that are too rough on the skin. Gloves are a fun way to exfoliate using any cleanser as they can be used on the face (gently) or the entire body.
Salt and sugar	A wonderful mechanical exfoliant in scrubs. Use gently in circular motions. Do not actually "scrub" your body of face with them.
Finely ground grains, beads, baking soda, sand	Many products contain different exfoliating ingredients. Be gentle with these ingredients as they can be too rough for sensitive skin.

HOW TO EXFOLIATE AND
HOW OFTEN TO DO IT

Generally exfoliating one to three times per week is best. This depends on skin sensitivity and skin type. For those with sensitive skin, exfoliating once a week may be all that you can do without sending your skin out of balance. For those with dry skin, be sure to use an exfoliating method that does not dry out your skin.

Gently massage exfoliants into the skin, taking your time. If a product irritates your skin, stop using it. Use a good serum and moisturizer after you have exfoliated. Begin with a simple product, such as a sugar scrub.

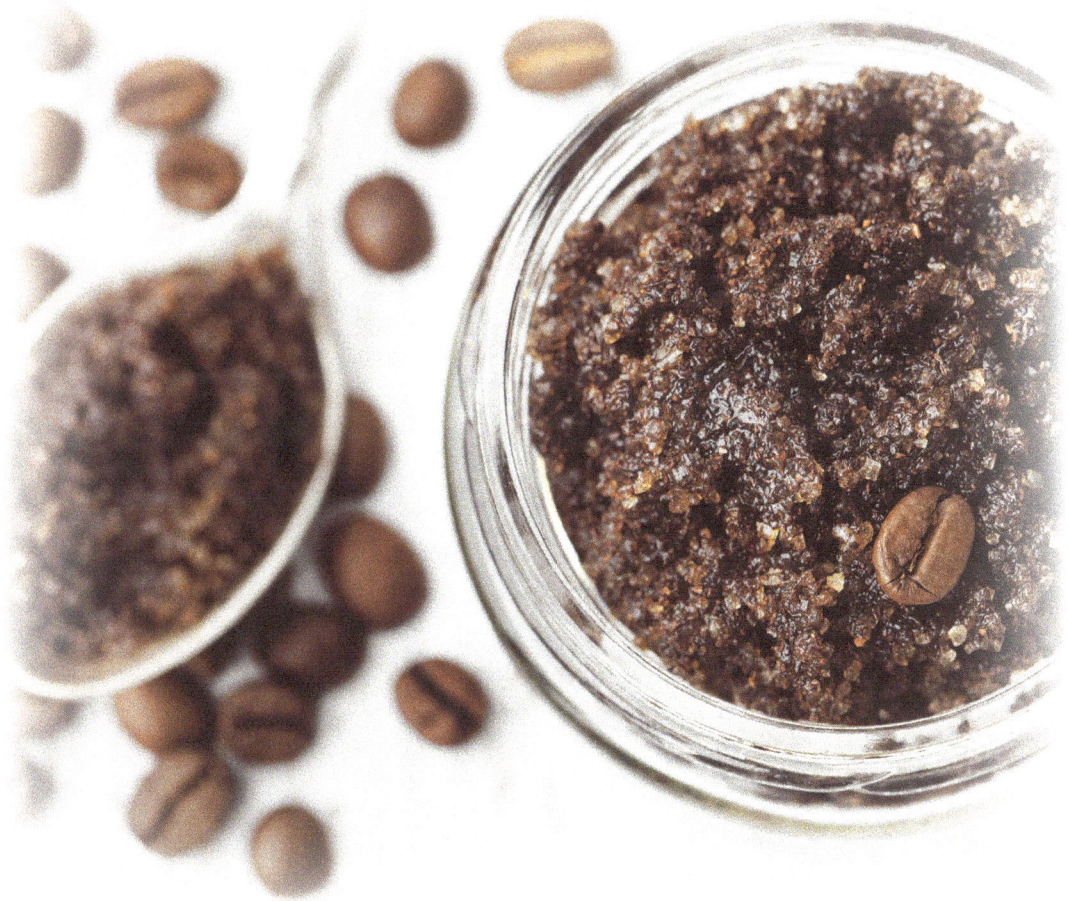

CINNAMON-COFFEE BODY SCRUB

Makes 6 ounces

Coffee can be a great ingredient to use as a natural exfoliant. The caffeine in coffee and the stimulant from cinnamon have been known to diminish the appearance of cellulite and tighten and tone your skin. Coffee grounds can also act as an excellent exfoliant when gently rolled over the skin. This scrub is intended to stick to the skin for maximum benefits. Because of that, you will want to rinse your body thoroughly after application. Get your skin glowing for summer with this simple coffee scrub.

    1 tablespoon finely ground (unused) coffee

    ½ cup pure cane sugar

    1 tablespoon olive oil

    2 tablespoons apricot oil

    1 teaspoon molasses

    1 teaspoon ground cinnamon

    ½ teaspoon almond extract

Combine all ingredients and store in a container with a lid.

In the shower, gently roll a couple of tablespoons of the scrub all over your body. (This recipe is not intended for the face.) Coat the skin and let the scrub sit for a minute or so. Rinse thoroughly. Your skin will feel invigorated and amazingly smooth after your shower. Do not use on damaged or irritated skin.

Caution: Be careful as this scrub can leave your shower or tub a bit slippery.

When to Discard: about 1 month

COCONUT-LEMON SUGAR SCRUB

Makes 8 ounces

1 cup pure white sugar

1 tablespoon raw honey

1½ tablespoons coconut oil

2 tablespoons 100% lemon juice

Combine all ingredients and store in a container with a lid.

The consistency should be a nice, thick paste. Use on your face and body a couple of times a week to exfoliate skin.

Caution: Be careful as this scrub can leave your shower or tub a bit slippery.

When to Discard: about 1 month

BROWN-SUGAR BODY SCRUB

Makes 4 ounces

½ cup of brown sugar

½ tablespoon of raw honey

2 tablespoons of almond oil, jojoba oil, or olive oil

3–5 drops of lemon or vanilla essential oil (optional)

Mix ingredients thoroughly in a bowl, then transfer and store in a container with a lid.

Use the scrub all over your body and rinse well with warm water. This is a great scrub for hands and feet as well. It is also preferred by those who have oily skin. Not recommended for acne-prone skin.

Caution: Be careful as this scrub can leave your shower or tub a bit slippery.

When to Discard: about 1 month

HONEY-WALNUT BODY POLISH

Makes 5 ounces

½ cup pure cane sugar

¼ cup walnut oil

2 teaspoons raw honey

1 tablespoon finely ground walnuts (the meat, not the shell)

Combine all ingredients and store in a container with a lid.

Use a couple of times a week in the shower as a body polish. This recipe can also be used as a hand scrub. Rinse thoroughly.

When to Discard: about 1 month

OIL-BALANCING SEA-SALT SCRUB

Makes 8 ounces

1 cup sea salt

2½ tablespoons avocado oil or grapeseed oil

1 tablespoon raw unfiltered honey

1 tablespoon pure lemon juice

½ tablespoon witch hazel

5 drops frankincense essential oil (optional)

Combine all ingredients in a bowl and transfer to a jar or container with a lid.

While in the shower, gently roll the scrub over your skin. This can be gently used on the face for those with oily skin. It is great body scrub for all skin types. Rinse thoroughly.

Caution: Be careful as this scrub can leave your shower or tub a bit slippery.

When to Discard: about 1 month

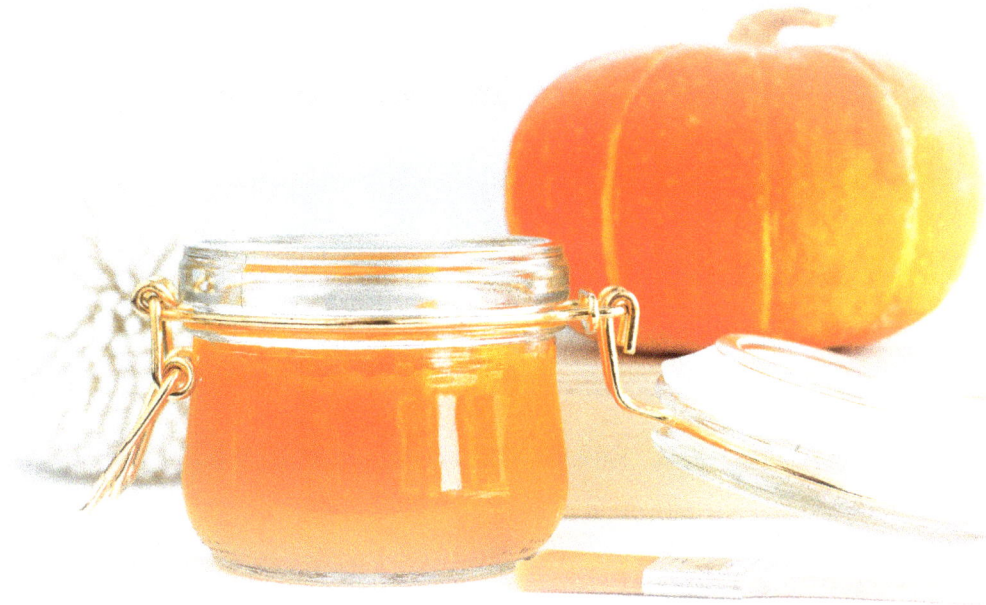

THE BENEFITS OF PUMPKIN

There are so many reasons to love pumpkin, and it is no surprise it is so popular during fall. Pumpkin is very low in calories and contains no saturated fats or cholesterol. It is rich in dietary fiber, antioxidants, minerals, and vitamins, and it can be beneficial for weight loss and diet control. Pumpkin has many antioxidant vitamins such as vitamins A, C, and E, and it is rich in minerals like copper, calcium, potassium, and phosphorus. Pumpkin is also an excellent source of beta-carotene, which is a carotenoid compound responsible for giving fruits and vegetables their orange pigment. It is considered a powerful antioxidant and is believed to help protect against cancer and aging.

Anything you put inside your body will show on the outside. Eating nutrient-dense foods will ultimately show up as beautiful skin, but it also helps to put these amazing nutrients directly on the skin's surface. Pumpkin is packed with enzymes and alpha hydroxy acids (AHAs). With this combination you will find increased cell turnover and brighter, smoother skin. Pumpkin's components can help even out skin tone and give it a beautiful glow.

Pumpkin can also be very hydrating for the skin. Although it's an amazing natural exfoliant, this squash does not leave your face dry. Pumpkin can penetrate deep into the skin when used topically but it is still gentle enough for sensitive skin. The vitamin A and vitamin C in pumpkin will help soften and smooth the skin while boosting collagen production to prevent signs of aging.

NOURISHING PUMPKIN BODY SCRUB

Makes 8 ounces

   1 cup sugar

   ½ cup pure pumpkin, pureed*

   ¼ cup coconut oil (not fractionated)

   1 tablespoon raw honey

Combine all ingredients and store in a plastic container with a lid.

Toward the end of your shower, apply body scrub gently to your body using circular motions. Leave it on for a few minutes if you prefer a deeper cleanse. Rinse thoroughly.

This scrub is very mild and nourishing for the skin. It is gentle enough to use daily. If you prefer a more intense scrub, increase sugar to your consistency preference.

Raw pumpkin contains vitamins and enzymes that are very beneficial for the skin. You can use raw, pureed pumpkin, but if you don't want to use the food processor or worry about a big mess, canned pumpkin (100 percent pure) will work just fine. If you do use raw pumpkin, just know that it can be more intense on the skin because of the active enzymes.

Caution: Be careful as this scrub can leave your shower or tub a bit slippery.

When to Discard: about 1 month

SWEET RED BODY SCRUB

Makes 16 ounces

- 1½ cups pure cane sugar

- ½ cup pink Himalayan salt, finely ground

- 2 tablespoons aloe vera juice

- ½ tablespoon beetroot powder

- 2 teaspoons almond oil

- ½ teaspoon almond extract

- 10 drops vanilla essential oil

Combine sugar and salt and mix well. Add remaining ingredients. Pour into two 8-ounce containers with a sealable lid.

Use a couple times a week. Because of its color, Sweet Red Body Scrub makes a wonderful Valentine's Day gift.

Caution: Be careful as this scrub can leave your shower or tub a bit slippery.

When to Discard: about 1 month

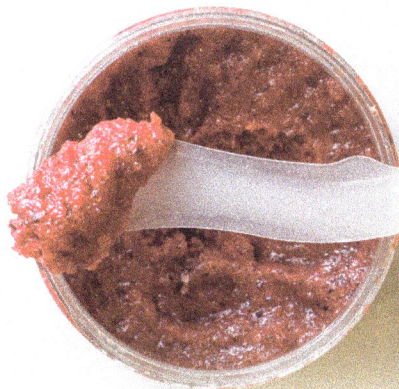

PROTECTIVE-DEFENSE SALT SCRUB

Makes 5 ounces

This pretty-smelling, exfoliating salt scrub is for your hands. Keep it in an elegant glass container next to the sink for family and guests. The added bonus is that this cleansing scrub contains antibacterial essential oils, which can help protect you during cold and flu season. An added bonus: kids love washing their hands with this fun salt scrub.

½ cup Epsom salts

1 tablespoon Dead Sea salt

1 tablespoon pink Himalayan salt

½ teaspoon almond oil

2 drops eucalyptus essential oil

3 drops wild orange essential oil

1 drop clove essential oil

Combine all ingredients. Store in a pretty jar with a lid or in an open bowl by your sink. Having a little spoon to take out a scoop at a time works best.

Apply a scoop (about 1½ teaspoons) to wet hands and massage thoroughly. Rinse off salts and finish with a nourishing lotion or body butter (See Lavender Body Butter on page 117).

When to Discard: about 6 months

CHAPTER 8

Make Your Own

FACIAL MASKS

Facial masks are so easy to make, *and* they give amazing results. In addition, you can save a lot of money by making your own facial masks at home. Fresh ingredients are often more effective at treating the skin than a professional mask. Here are a few of my favorite ingredients for homemade facial masks.

Avocado	Great moisturizer, high in vitamin B and potassium. Nourishing for the skin and gives your face a glow.
Banana	Skin softening and nourishing. Wonderful for dry skin. High in vitamin C and potassium.
Clay	Great for oily and acne-prone skin. Draws out impurities and softens skin.
Honey	Firms skin and helps relieve dryness. Helps with breakouts and also balances skin.

Oats	Anti-inflammatory, calming, and helps with hydration. Great for sensitive skin.
Pineapple	High in vitamin C and bromelain, an enzyme that softens skin and can minimize inflammation.
Pomegranate	High in antioxidants and vitamin C. Has anti-aging properties.
Pumpkin	Anti-aging and antioxidant. Packed with vitamins A and C. Also hydrates and softens skin.
Sugar	Both white and brown sugar help exfoliate the skin. It smoothes and softens, giving your face a nice glow.
Turmeric	Brightening and calming. A wonderful ingredient to calm acne and revitalize dull skin.
Yogurt	Contains lactic acid, which helps even out skin tone and sloughs off dead skin cells, helping with skin turnover.

Do not hesitate to play with various ingredients for masks. It is much more fun to be creative. You can mix different ingredients and come up with your own concoctions, depending on what your skin needs.

A WORD ON MANGO

Avoid using mango in your own skin-care masks. Mango skins contain a skin-irritating compound that's also in poison ivy, so this tropical fruit is not the best choice for a do-it-yourself mask.

HONEY-OAT HYDRATING MASK

Makes enough for one use

> 1 tablespoon of honey
>
> 1 teaspoon oil (almond, grapeseed, jojoba, or olive)
>
> ½ teaspoon ground oats or oat flour (optional)

Make a simple mask by mixing honey with a little bit of oil. If you add ground oats to the mask, it can help reduce redness and irritated skin.

Mix your mask and apply to your face. Leave on for approximately 5 minutes. Rinse off completely, and finish with a high-quality night cream.

When to Discard: Use up immediately; do not store

TURMERIC'S TRADITIONAL ROOTS

I am obsessed with turmeric because it is great for the body and great for the skin. In many parts of India, the spice made from the turmeric root is healing and ceremonial. Turmeric is traditionally used as an essential part of beauty routines. When applied to the skin as a paste or a face mask, it can help treat acne, eczema, and rosacea, and it adds a glow to the skin.

The anti-inflammatory and antioxidant properties of turmeric are both important for treating skin conditions. Facial masks containing turmeric can calm blemishes and heal the skin. For eczema, turmeric can reduce inflammation and redness. When rosacea sufferers use turmeric masks, tiny pimples and redness associated with flareups can be reduced. Regular use of turmeric masks may also soften the appearance of wrinkles and fine lines.

Turmeric root is packed with nutrients and is popular in Indian cooking, and for centuries it has been used in wedding ceremonies. One of the most important ceremonies of an Indian wedding is the *haldi*, or *ubtan*, ceremony when the bride and groom prepare for their wedding by applying a traditional turmeric paste to their faces and bodies.

Family haldi recipes are traditional and can differ, but commonly it is a mixture of turmeric, sandalwood powder or some type of flour, and rose water or water. The paste is then applied by their relatives to the bride's and groom's face, neck, hands, and feet. The ceremony is accompanied by traditional songs and dances and is a joyous pre-wedding ritual. Traditionally, it was done separately, but in current times many couples choose to share the joyous occasion.

Turmeric is known to have properties that leave the skin fair and glowing. Additionally, regular use of turmeric masks can help eliminate fine facial hair. Turmeric can also exfoliate and detoxify the skin. The haldi ceremony is like an in-home beautification process before the wedding, but we can mimic this tradition and get the benefits anytime.

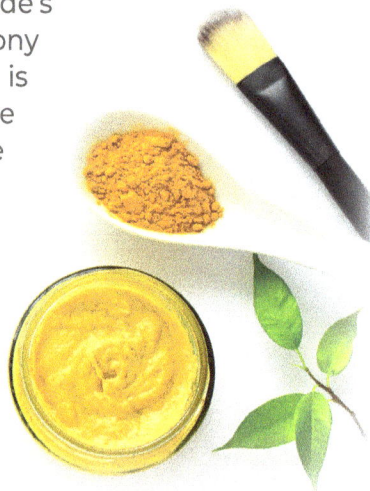

BRIGHTENING TURMERIC GLOW MASK

Makes enough for one use

- ½ teaspoon ground turmeric*
- ½ teaspoon grapeseed oil or almond oil
- ½ teaspoon raw honey
- ¼ teaspoon rice flour (optional)

Combine all ingredients and mix well.

Cleanse face, if needed. Apply a thin layer of turmeric mask all over face, avoiding brows and hairline. Wash hands immediately. Let mask sit on the skin for about 5 minutes. Rinse face thoroughly with a colored washcloth (not white). Proceed with your normal skin-care routine.

Be careful not to get any of the mask mixture on countertops or clothing as turmeric stains easily. It usually washes out, but just use caution.

When to Discard: use immediately, do not store

NOURISHING TURMERIC TRADITIONAL MASK

Makes enough for one use

½ teaspoon ground turmeric*

¼ teaspoon raw honey

1 tablespoon whole-wheat flour

2½ teaspoons milk**

1 drop sandalwood essential oil

Combine all ingredients and mix well.

Cleanse face, if needed. Apply a thin layer of turmeric mask all over face, avoiding brows and hairline. Wash hands immediately. Let mask sit on the skin for about 5 minutes. Rinse face thoroughly. It is best to rinse off this mask in the shower because it can be thick and messy. Use a colored washcloth, not white. Proceed with your normal skin-care routine.

* Be careful not to get any of the mask mixture on countertops or clothing, as turmeric stains easily. It usually washes out, but use caution.

** Can use a milk substitute, such as almond milk.

When to Discard: Use immediately; do not store.

DEEP-CLEANSING CLAY MASK

Makes enough for one use

Use all-natural calcium bentonite (green) clay, available at most local health-food stores.

> 1 tablespoon bentonite clay
>
> 1 tablespoon apple cider vinegar (or water for sensitive skin)

Combine ingredients in a nonmetal container. The consistency should be like thick mud.

This mask is strong smelling and strong acting. It can make the face tingle, and the apple cider vinegar (see page 197 to make your own) can make your eyes water because the scent is so pungent. For those with oily skin, this is a great mask.

Apply about a ⅛ to ¼ inch layer all over face, avoiding eyes. Do *not* allow the mask to completely harden. Wait until it has started to dry but is still sticky. This means it has begun to pull impurities out of the skin. If you let it get too dry you risk dehydrating the skin and causing an imbalance. Rinse with warm water and apply your usual facial moisturizer. Slight redness may temporarily occur.

When to Discard: Use immediately; do not store.

SWEET BANANA MOISTURE MASK

Makes enough for one use

1 overripe banana   1 tablespoon honey

Mash a very ripe banana and add about a tablespoon of honey to make a paste.

Apply directly to skin. Let it sit a few minutes, then rinse off. This mask works well if you are about to take a shower. Keep the mask on your skin for about five minutes while you're in the shower, allowing the steam to help open the pores. It causes less mess this way.

When to Discard: Use immediately; do not store.

KID-FRIENDLY MOISTURIZING MASK

Makes enough for one use

This wonderful face mask is great for kids of all ages. It is extremely moisturizing and gentle, so it works well for dry or dehydrated skin. Additionally, it can help relieve eczema-prone skin.

1 tablespoon raw, organic coconut oil

1 tablespoon honey

1 tablespoon oat flour

Combine all ingredients.

Apply gently to your child's skin; if they are older they might enjoy doing it themselves. Leave on about 3–5 minutes. Rinse thoroughly.

When to Discard: Use immediately; do not store.

ACTIVATED CHARCOAL BENEFITS

Activated charcoal is an amazing addition to natural skin care. It is normally taken as a dietary supplement as a safe remedy for bloating and upset stomach. Used in emergency trauma centers across the world, activated charcoal has been proven effective for removing ingested toxins. Activated charcoal is very porous and is able to trap toxins, bacteria, dirt, and chemicals. In skin care, it absorbs dirt from the pores and bacteria from blemishes. This helps purify and detoxify the skin. Charcoal clearing masks can be beneficial for oily skin, breakouts, and acne.

Activated charcoal is *not* the same as charcoal in your barbecue grill, which is loaded with toxins and chemicals and is not safe to consume.

Activated charcoal is a substance made from bone char, coconut shells, petroleum, and/or coal. The substance is then oxidized using steam or air, at high temperatures. This process gives it a medicinal property and makes it very porous so that it is able to absorb toxins. It is truly an amazing ingredient to have on hand for skin care. A more natural form of activated charcoal, such as one made from coconut shells, is best.

There are many charcoal masks currently on the market, that can be very hard on the skin. These are the black peel-off masks you may have seen on social media. They are extremely sticky, with harsh ingredients. Removing the masks can, in some cases, cause damage to the skin as they do not remove easily. Try a more gentle charcoal mask, like the recipe listed in this section.

ACTIVATED CHARCOAL
SKIN-CLEARING MASK

Makes enough for one use

1 capsule of activated charcoal *

2 teaspoons aloe vera gel

3 drops tea tree essential oil **

Break open the charcoal capsule and combine it with the other ingredients in a small container. Mix well. Gently massage onto cleansed skin, avoiding the eye and mouth areas. Leave on your skin for 3–5 minutes and rinse thoroughly.

* This mask is black in color. Activated charcoal can stain grout and fabrics. It can also temporarily dye your hairline or eyebrows if you have light-colored hair. Protect counters and clothing from staining as well.

** If your skin is very sensitive, use only 1 drop of tea tree essential oil—or avoid altogether.

When to Discard: Use immediately; do not store.

CHOCOLATE MUD MASK

Makes enough for one use

This recipe is wonderful for dry or damaged skin and it smells delicious!

- 2 tablespoons plain yogurt

- 1 teaspoon cocoa powder

- ¼ ripe banana, mashed

- 1 teaspoon honey

- 1 teaspoon lemon juice

Combine all ingredients and mix thoroughly. If you want this mask to be super-smooth, use a blender to make it nice and creamy.

Apply the mask to your skin using circular motions. Let it sit on the skin for 4–6 minutes, then rinse thoroughly. Continue with your normal skin-care routine.

When to Discard: Use immediately; do not store.

EXFOLIATING GINGERBREAD POWDER MASK

Makes one 5-ounce powder mix

This mask is definitely a fall favorite. It smells just like gingerbread cookies!

2 tablespoons fine sugar	½ teaspoon pumpkin-pie spice
1 tablespoon brown sugar	⅛ teaspoon almond extract
1 tablespoon oat flour	3 drops vanilla essential oil
1 tablespoon bentonite clay	2 drops benzoin essential oil

Combine all ingredients and mix well. Store in a small container with a lid until needed.

Use 1 teaspoon of powder at a time and mix with 1 teaspoon of liquid (you can use water, milk, yogurt, or coconut water) to make a mask.

Cleanse your face, if needed. Apply a thin layer of the gingerbread mask all over your face, avoiding brows and hairline. Let the mask sit on the skin for about 5 minutes. Rinse your face thoroughly with a colored washcloth (not white). Proceed with your normal skin-care routine.

When to Discard: Powder will last about 3 months

CLARIFYING ROSE CLAY MASK

Makes enough for one use

- 1 teaspoon oat flour

- 1 teaspoon bentonite-clay powder

- ¼ teaspoon rose powder (optional)

- 1 teaspoon aloe vera gel

- 1 teaspoon rose hydrosol or 1 teaspoon aloe vera juice (see page 153)

- 2 drops grapefruit (or a rose blend) essential oil

Combine dry ingredients first, then add aloe, hydrosol, and essential oils. Mix ingredients thoroughly. Apply to skin using circular motions. Let sit on the skin for 4–6 minutes, then rinse thoroughly. Continue your normal skin-care routine.

When to Discard: Use immediately; do not store.

WHAT IS DIATOMACEOUS EARTH?

Diatomaceous earth, sometimes called DE or diatomite, is fossilized sedimentary rock that easily crumbles into a powder. Each particle is very fine, less than a millimeter in size. These tiny, fossilized aquatic organisms are mined in areas containing fossilized sediment, where bodies of water once existed. The skeletons of these little, deceased organisms are made of a natural substance called silica.

Silica makes up about 26 percent of the Earth's crust. Different forms of silica include sand, mica, clay, emerald, quartz, feldspar, and glass. This fine powder has an abrasive texture because of the sharp, skeletal remains.

Josh Axe, DC, DNM, CNS, a well-known doctor of natural medicine, author, and nutritionist, states that diatomaceous earth works like a natural detoxifying agent within the body, killing parasites and viruses that can contribute to illnesses, while also helping to clean the blood. Additionally, a study published in the *American Journal of Clinical Nutrition* found that silica can assist in the elimination of heavy metals, such as aluminum, from the body. Some people take food-grade diatomaceous earth as a dietary supplement for a detoxifying cleanse.

Diatomaceous earth is used in cleaners, natural farm or garden pesticides, and skin-care products. When treating the skin, DE can be used in a mask or scrub to help pull toxins from the skin. Because of its natural exfoliating ability, it will leave behind clean, soft, polished skin.

Always use food-grade diatomaceous earth, as many DE products are mixed with other chemicals for various uses. You can find powdered, food-grade diatomaceous earth in health food stores or online.

FOAMING TURMERIC EXFOLIATING MASK

Makes enough for one use

¼ teaspoon turmeric powder*

1 tablespoon baking soda

½ tablespoon citric-acid powder

¼ teaspoon diatomaceous earth

water

Combine all dry ingredients and mix well. Add a few drops of water until the mixture foams up to form a foamy, paste-like consistency.

Cleanse your face, if needed. Apply a thin layer of the foaming mask all over your face, avoiding brows and hairline. Wash your hands immediately so the turmeric does not tint your hands or fingernails. Let the mask remain on the skin for about 5 minutes, then rinse your face thoroughly with a colored washcloth (not white). Proceed with your normal skin-care routine, being sure to apply moisturizer afterward as this mask can be drying to the skin.

* Be careful not to get any of the mask mixture on countertops or clothing as turmeric can stain easily. It usually washes out, but just use caution.

When to Discard: Use immediately; do not store.

CHAPTER 9

A FACIAL SERUM

Serums are a great way to apply vitamins and nutrients to your skin. Serums go on before your moisturizer so that they absorb more readily into the skin. Vitamins nourish the skin and help maintain its function. Certain vitamins, specifically A, C, and E and folic acid, are powerful antioxidants. Many of these nutrients are not produced by the body, so they must be consumed through diet or supplementation. Vitamins C and E are a couple of my favorite vitamins because they offer the fastest and most noticeable results in skin-care.

Antioxidants, Free Radicals, and the Skin

Antioxidants are complex molecules that help protect cells from damage by breaking down free radical chain reactions. Because of that, when antioxidants are applied to the skin, it helps to reverse the effects of sun damage.

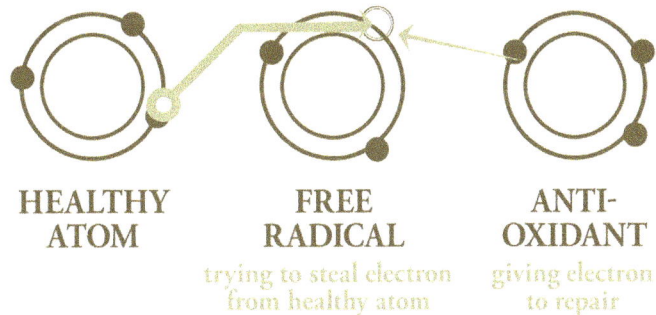

HEALTHY ATOM

FREE RADICAL
trying to steal electron from healthy atom

ANTI-OXIDANT
giving electron to repair

Free radicals are unstable atoms that enter into a destructive chemical bond with organic substances such as proteins. This results in oxidation. One example of oxidation in nature is when an apple or avocado turns brown after being cut. When you apply lemon juice onto the cut apple or avocado, the browning is minimal. The same concept applies when you put vitamin C on your skin. For free radicals to become more stable, they will take electrons from other atoms. This can cause diseases or signs of aging. That is where antioxidants are helpful.

As you can see, antioxidants are extremely important for overall health and can slow the aging process. One important thing to keep in mind when using citrus fruits and powdered or liquid vitamin C in your products is that they can cause sun sensitivity. Therefore, avoid being in the sun while wearing products that are high in vitamin C. Products containing large quantities of citrus extracts and oils should be applied primarily at bedtime.

Beneficial Antioxidants for the Skin	
Vitamin A	Both retinol and retinoid are derived from vitamin A but can often be synthetic or animal byproducts. These products are widely used by dermatologists and skin-care professionals to treat damaged skin, acne, or fine lines and wrinkles. Some natural alternatives are rosehip seed oil, carrots, and papaya.
Vitamin C	This important antioxidant is a key component in collagen synthesis. Vitamin C also plays a role in wound healing and inflammation. When free radicals break down collagen, skin fibers lose elasticity, and wrinkling begins to occur. One of the best ways to deliver vitamins to your skin is through topical creams. The other is by eating fruits and vegetables. Lemons and other citrus fruits are a great source of vitamin C.
Vitamin E	Vitamin E, also known as tocopherol, is one of the most essential antioxidants. The application of vitamin E to the skin has been shown to help boost collagen and reduce sun damage. Some studies show that approximately 80 percent of the signs of aging are caused by sun damage. There is evidence that vitamins C and E are more powerful when applied together.

SIMPLY HYDRATING NIGHT SERUM

Makes 1 ounce

This combination of oils is a wonderful serum for mature or dry skin, and it helps to reverse damage and hydrate the skin.

> 1 tablespoon pure argan oil
>
> 1 tablespoon pure rosehip seed oil
>
> 5–8 drops frankincense essential oil
>
> 3–5 drops lavender essential oil

Mix oils together. Using a funnel, pour the serum into a 1 ounce, dark-colored bottle with a glass dropper. Squeeze a quarter-dropper onto your hands and evenly distribute among your fingertips. Massage onto clean face and décolletage.

When to Discard: 6 months to a year, depending on the shelf life of the oils

GLOWING-SKIN OIL SERUM

Makes 2 ounces

1 tablespoon pure argan oil

1 tablespoon grapeseed oil

1 tablespoon pure rosehip seed oil

1 tablespoon almond oil

½ teaspoon pomegranate oil (optional)

½ dropper white willow bark tincture*

5 drops frankincense essential oil

6 drops lavender essential oil

4 drops ylang ylang

2 drops cedarwood

Mix oils together, and use a funnel to pour the serum into a 2 ounce, dark-colored glass dropper bottle. Squeeze a quarter dropper onto your hands and evenly distribute among your fingertips. Massage onto clean face and décolletage.

See page 158 if you want to make your own White Willow Bark Tincture.

When to Discard: 6 months to a year, depending on the shelf life of the oils

INTENSELY GREEN NIGHT SERUM

Makes 2 ounces

> 1 tablespoon cold-pressed flaxseed oil
>
> 1 tablespoon almond oil
>
> 1 tablespoon argan oil
>
> 1 tablespoon rosehip seed oil
>
> ½ tablespoon chlorophyll powder or infused oil
>
> ⅛ teaspoon sea buckthorn oil

Use a funnel to pour all ingredients into a glass dropper bottle. (Chlorophyll can easily turn a serum rancid, so use this serum up quickly.)

Use a quarter to half dropper every evening. Apply to your hands and rub them together before applying to your entire face and décolletage. Leave the serum on overnight and rinse off in the morning.

When to Discard: about 1 month

MOISTURIZING ROSE OIL SERUM

Makes 2 ounces

1 tablespoon rosehip seed oil

⅛ teaspoon vitamin E oil

1 tablespoon apricot oil

1 tablespoon grapeseed oil

1 tablespoon fractionated coconut oil

5 drops rose essential oil*

Use a funnel to pour all ingredients into a glass dropper bottle. Use a half dropper every evening. Apply to your hands and rub them together before applying to your entire face and décolletage. Leave on overnight and rinse off in the morning.

Most rose essential oil is blended with another oil. Pure rose essential oil is extremely expensive and you would only need one drop versus five of the blended.

When to Discard: 6 months to a year, depending on the shelf life of the oils

VITAMIN C BOOST SERUM

Makes 2 ounces

Vitamin C facial serums are very popular and for good reason. Everyone loves adding a few extra vitamins to their skin. Vitamin C helps brighten the skin and eliminate fine lines. It can be very effective as a treatment for dull, dehydrated skin. Your skin cells regenerate the most while you sleep, so include this amazing vitamin C serum in your regular routine each evening. Vitamin C powder is also known as ascorbic acid, which is often sold in health food stores.

2 tablespoons grapeseed oil	½ teaspoon castor oil
1 teaspoon apricot oil	½ teaspoon avocado oil
1 tablespoon glycerine	4 drops frankincense essential oil
¼ teaspoon powdered vitamin C	6 drops orange or bergamot essential oil

Combine glycerine and powdered vitamin C first, whisking together until well blended. Combine the glycerine mixture with other ingredients. With a small funnel, pour the serum into a 2 ounce glass dropper bottle.

Use about a half dropper every evening. First apply it to your hands and rub them together before spreading the serum to your entire face and décolletage. Leave on overnight and rinse off in the morning. The glycerine tends to settle at the bottom so shake well before each use.

When to Discard: 6 months to a year, depending on shelf life of oils

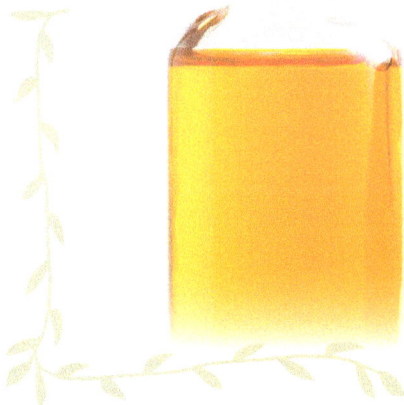

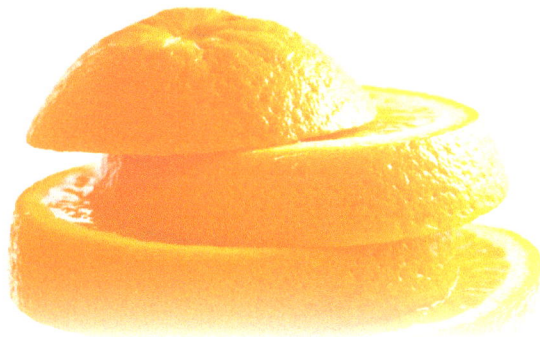

COFFEE & GREEN TEA BALANCING SERUM

Makes 2 ounces

Both coffee and green tea contain caffeine, which can help stimulate the skin. They also contain antioxidants that can help protect the skin and slow signs of aging. This facial serum helps fight acne, discoloration, and puffiness, and it makes the skin nice and smooth. Lemon is great for brightening, and chamomile calms the skin, which can help with breakouts.

¼ cup Green Tea & Coffee Infused Oil*

10 drops lemon essential oil

10 drops chamomile essential oil

Add the lemon and chamomile essential oils to the infused oil mixture, and transfer into a 2 ounce glass dropper bottle or two 1 ounce glass dropper bottles. Every evening put about a half dropper amount into the palm of your hands. Rub your hands together and apply the serum evenly all over your face and décolletage.

* See page 155 for instructions on how to make Green Tea & Coffee Infused Oil.

When to Discard: 6 months to a year depending on shelf life of oils

BEARD OIL DUO-SERUM FOR MEN

Makes 8 ounces

Beard oil can change an unruly beard into a soft, tamable one. My husband grows a beard every year for hunting season. I love the way it looks, but before beard oil, I did not like the way his beard felt against my skin. I have very sensitive skin, and his beard was prickly, even after it was completely grown out.

Because of that, I began making beard oil anytime he chose to grow a beard. Of course, as an esthetician, I could not stop there: I also wanted a serum that was great for his skin. So this recipe is different from your typical beard oil because it also acts as an oil facial serum.

The essential oils in this recipe are very healing, and the serum has an earthy smell. This recipe makes a large batch—about three or four 2 ounce glass dropper bottles.

¼ cup grapeseed oil

⅛ cup apricot oil

1 tablespoon rosehip seed oil

1 tablespoon jojoba

¼ teaspoon argan oil

8–10 drops frankincense essential oil

8–10 drops tea tree essential oil

7–9 drops peppermint essential oil

4–6 drops vetiver essential oil

Combine all ingredients, and pour into two 4 ounce amber colored glass dropper bottles.

Apply about a half dropper of beard oil into the palm of your hand and rub hands together, distributing evenly. It is best to massage the oil into the beard first, from the follicle to the ends of the beard.

Massage the remaining beard oil all over your face. It takes a few minutes for the beard oil to absorb into the skin because it is so moisturizing.

This recipe makes a great gift because it makes a large batch and is so easy to personalize.

When to Discard: 6 months to a year depending on shelf life of oils

HAIR-STIMULATING BEARD OIL

Makes 2 ounces

Rosemary and peppermint both stimulate hair follicles and can encourage hair growth. This is a great formula for men who have a hard time getting their facial hair to grow in evenly.

> 1 tablespoon grapeseed oil
>
> 1 tablespoon olive oil
>
> 1 tablespoon jojoba oil
>
> 1 tablespoon fractionated coconut oil
>
> 5 drops peppermint essential oil
>
> 5 drops rosemary essential oil

Combine all ingredients and pour into a 2 ounce dropper bottle. Apply about a half dropper of beard oil into the palm of your hand and rub your hands together, distributing evenly. It is best to massage beard oil into the beard first, from the follicle to the ends of the beard.

When to Discard: 6 months to a year depending on shelf life of oils

CHAPTER 10

Caring for the Skin

AROUND YOUR EYES

The eyes are the most delicate area of the face and most susceptible to fine lines, puffiness and dryness. For that reason, I like to give them special attention. The skin below the eyes is thinner and therefore prone to wrinkles. The area around the eyes lacks both muscle and soft tissue, like fat, making it harder to keep a youthful appearance. Additionally, dark circles and puffiness can be present as a result of sleepless nights, poor diet, and stress.

"I'm laughing on the inside so I don't get wrinkles."

—Unknown

Some store-bought eye creams contain harsh ingredients and preservatives that can actually make dryness and inflammation worse around the eyes. The last thing you want is to dry out the areas around your eyes, as that leads to wrinkling of the skin. A more natural product that increases hydration will give you better results.

REJUVENATING EYE SERUM

Makes enough for two 10 ml. roller bottles

2 tablespoons Green Tea & Coffee Infused Oil*

1/8 teaspoon rosehip seed oil

1/8 teaspoon castor oil

1/8 teaspoon liquid C ** (optional)

1/2 dropper sea buckthorn oil

5 drops frankincense essential oil

5 drops lavender essential oil

3 drops chamomile essential oil (optional)

Combine all ingredients, and pour into either a roller ball bottle or a 1 ounce dropper bottle.

Gently shake before each use. Roll this serum under your eyes every morning and evening.

* See page 155 for how to make Green Tea & Coffee Infused Oil. Can also use straight grapeseed oil if do not want an infused oil.

**Liquid C is available at most health food stores.

When to Discard: 6 months to a year, depending on shelf life of oils

HYDRATING-LEMON EYE MASK

Makes 8 small ½-ounce containers (for gifts) or a 4-ounce container

1/4 cup raw, unrefined coconut oil

2 teaspoons beeswax*

2 tablespoons castor oil

1 teaspoon jojoba oil or carrot seed oil

7 drops lemon essential oil

Combine all ingredients except the essential oil. Heat on very low temperature on your stovetop just until melted. Remove from heat and add the essential oil. Place in the refrigerator for about 10 to 15 minutes until the mask begins to set and achieves a gel-like consistency. Remove from the refrigerator and stir well. Pour into desired containers and let completely cool until you seal containers. (I like to use two 2 ounce glass containers with lids and give one away as a present.) Use every morning and evening by gently applying under and around eyes with fingertips.

* Use beeswax pastilles, wafers, or beads because they are so much easier to work with and measure than large chunks of beeswax.

When to Discard: about 2 months

GREEN TEA & COFFEE EYE CREAM

Makes 1 ounce

> 2 tablespoons Coffee & Green Tea Balancing Serum (page 86)
>
> 1 teaspoon beeswax*

Heat on very low temperature on stove until serum and beeswax are melted. Remove from heat. Put into small easy to use containers with a lid. Let cool several hours or let sit overnight. Do NOT seal your container until it has completely cooled. Use morning and evening, gently applying under and around eyes with fingertips.

* Use beeswax pastilles, wafers, or beads because they are so much easier to work with and measure than large chunks of beeswax.

When to Discard: about 6 months

EYE-MAKEUP REMOVER

Makes 5 ounces

Eye-makeup removers can be helpful with maintaining and hydrating your eyes. It seems unreasonable that there would be chemicals in store-bought eye-makeup removers but it is true. Thankfully, eye-makeup remover is extremely easy to make yourself because it contains simple ingredients and can save you money!

½ cup almond oil   5 drops lavender essential oil

⅛ cup pure witch hazel

Combine ingredients in a small container that has a pump or flip-cap. Shake gently before each use.

Apply to a cotton ball and gently wipe makeup from the eyes. Cleanse your face as usual.

When to Discard: about 6 months

SIMPLE EYE-MAKEUP REMOVER

Here's a super-simple way to remove eye-makeup in a pinch. Jojoba is hydrating and easy to use.

100% pure jojoba oil

Apply oil to a cotton ball, and gently wipe away makeup from the eyes. Cleanse your face as usual.

When to Discard: about a year depending on shelf life of oil

CHAPTER 11

How to Keep

YOUR LIPS PRETTY

One area that is often missed in skin care is the lips. Keeping them healthy and nourished makes our overall facial appearance all the better. Our lips take a lot of damage with extreme cold or dry weather. If left untreated, dehydrated lips can lead to cracking, which may be hard to heal. No one likes dealing with cracked, flaky lips. The DIY recipes in this chapter are geared toward replenishing moisture and repairing the delicate skin covering the lip area.

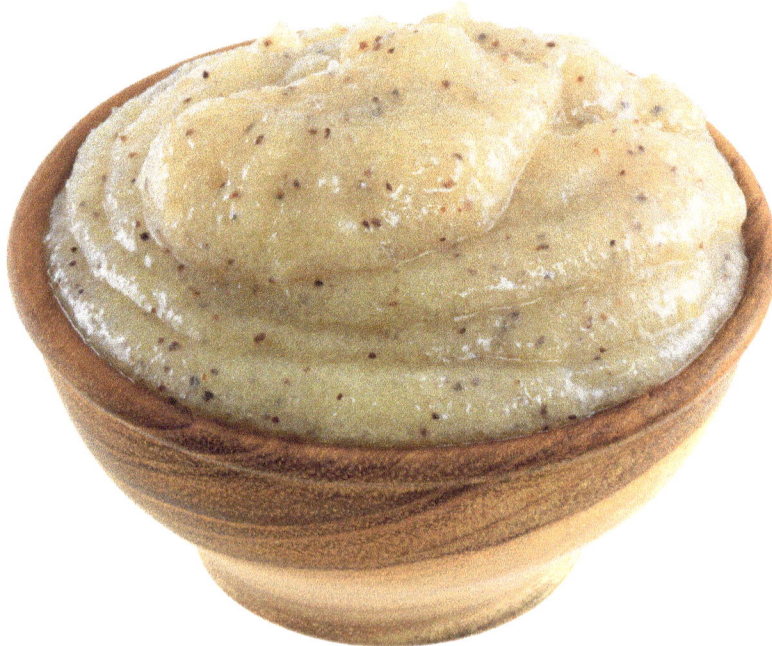

HONEY-CINNAMON
LIP PLUMPING SCRUB

Makes 1 ounce

Herbs and spices have amazing benefits for the skin. One spice I love for skin care is cinnamon, which brings circulation to the skin's surface. Alone, cinnamon can be too strong for the skin, but when mixed with a good oil it offers beautiful results, such as plumper lips. A lip scrub is really helpful for repairing dry, flaky skin on and around the mouth. This wonderful DIY recipe always leaves the lips feeling soft and smooth.

½ tablespoon sugar

1 teaspoon fractionated coconut oil

¼ teaspoon honey

¼ teaspoon cinnamon

3 drops vanilla extract

Mix ingredients thoroughly. Gently rub over lips in a circular motion. Leave on the lip area for 30 seconds to 1 minute. Rinse thoroughly and follow with a natural lip balm like the Fresh Peppermint Lip Balm recipe on page 96.

Leftover scrub can be saved in a little container for future use, if desired.

When to Discard: about a month

FRESH PEPPERMINT LIP BALM

Makes 10 lip balms

¼ cup coconut oil

1 tablespoon + 1 teaspoon of beeswax*

10 drops peppermint essential oil

Melt the coconut oil and beeswax together. Add the essential oils. Using an eye dropper, fill a container of your choice (empty Chapstick tubes or small lip gloss containers) and allow to completely cool before sealing.

* Use beeswax pastilles, wafers, or beads because they are so much easier to work with and measure than large chunks of beeswax.

When to Discard: about 3 months

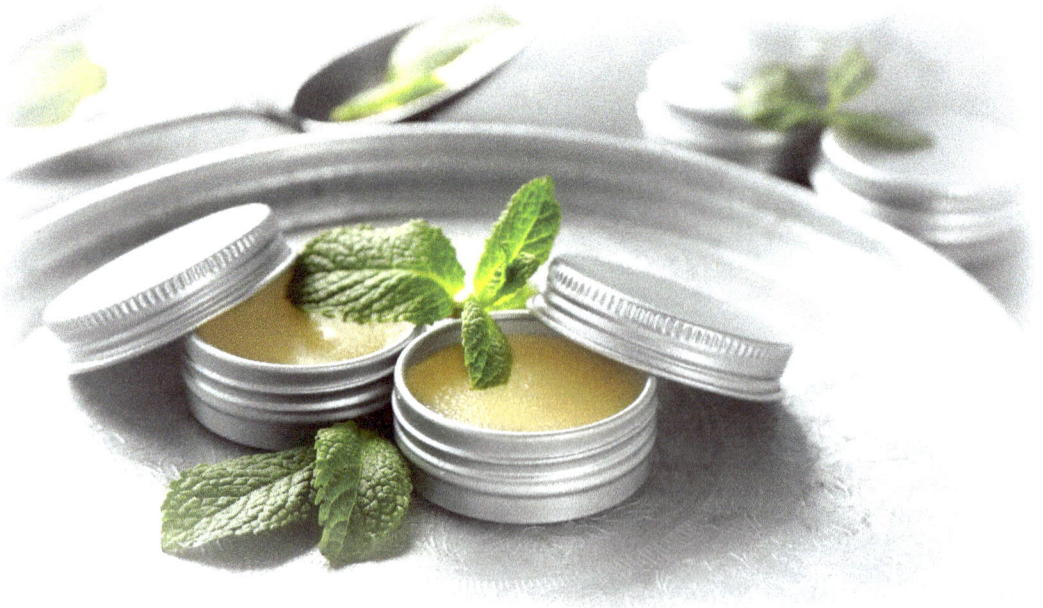

LOVELY LAVENDER LIP BALM

Makes 15 sticks

2 tablespoons cocoa butter*

1 tablespoon almond oil (infused with lavender if desired)

1 tablespoons castor oil

1 tablespoon + 1 teaspoon beeswax*

5 drops lavender essential oil

5 drops vanilla essential oil (optional)

Melt the coconut oil and beeswax together. Add the essential oils. Using an eye dropper, fill a container of your choice (empty Chapstick tubes or small lip gloss containers) and allow to completely cool before sealing.

Use beeswax pastilles, wafers, or beads because they are so much easier to work with and measure than large chunks of beeswax.

When to Discard: about 3 months

CHAPTER 12

Protecting Your Skin:

NATURAL MOISTURIZERS AND SUNSCREEN

An important step in your skin-care routine is protecting your skin. A good moisturizer will help lock in moisture and maintain a youthful appearance. Moisturizer can also help prevent breakouts by keeping the skin balanced. When your skin is hydrated, your oil glands are able to work normally. Letting your skin dry out could cause oil production to increase, which can clog pores and lead to unnecessary pimples.

By applying a nightly moisturizer, your serums are "locked in," so to speak. Protecting the skin is the final step in your skin-care routine—and it's a crucial one.

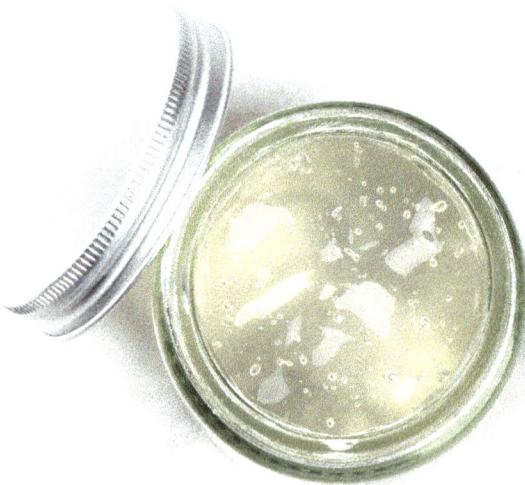

LIGHT ALOE FACIAL MOISTURIZER

Makes 2 ounces

> 2 tablespoons aloe vera gel
>
> 2 teaspoons raw, unrefined coconut oil
>
> ¼ teaspoon xanthan gum
>
> 2 drops frankincense essential oil (optional)

In a pot, slightly melt coconut oil and remove from heat. Add xanthan gum and mix well. Slowly add in aloe vera gel. Stir rapidly for several minutes until the moisturizer begins to gel. Add in essential oil, and stir well. Spoon the mixture in a sealable container that is easy to use, like an amber-colored glass jar or a Mason jar.

Apply this soothing moisturizer to your skin every evening at bedtime. You can also use this moisturizer during the day, but because it has a gel-like consistency, it tends to flake off a bit when you apply makeup.

When to Discard: about a month

COCONUT-VANILLA FACIAL CRÉME

Makes 1 ounce

1 tablespoon aloe vera gel

1 tablespoon raw, unrefined coconut oil

½ teaspoon vanilla extract

⅛ teaspoon xanthan gum

In a pot, slightly melt the coconut oil and remove from heat. Add xanthan gum and mix well. Slowly add in aloe vera gel and vanilla extract. Stir rapidly for several minutes until it begins to gel. Spoon the moisturizer into a sealable container that is easy to use, like an amber-colored glass jar or a Mason jar.

Apply this moisturizer to your skin every evening at bedtime. You can also use this moisturizer during the day, but because it has a gel-like consistency, it tends to flake off a bit when you apply makeup.

When to Discard: about a month

NICE & GENTLE SKIN OIL

Makes 6 ounces

When my son was a toddler, I had a hard time finding a lotion that did not irritate his skin. As a result, I decided to make him a moisturizing oil. Most lotions would cause an eczema-like rash on his skin. There were only a few products I tried that had better ingredients and seemed to be less irritating, but these brands were extremely expensive. Some of the petroleum-based products did help improve his skin. However, I did not like to use them because petroleum-based products are possibly carcinogenic and harmful.

After a lot of research—and some trial and error—I came up with this formula, which has worked wonders! As you can see, it is not a lotion but a skin oil. It works the same way, but it is thinner and coats and protects the skin. Skin oil is really easy to make and does not contain water, so it stays fresher for a longer period of time than lotion. This is my favorite recipe.

¼ cup pure almond oil*

¼ cup pure grapeseed oil

2 tablespoons castor oil

1 full dropper of sea buckthorn oil

Combine all ingredients thoroughly. Pour into a sealable container that is easy to use, like a bottle with a pump or an amber-colored glass bottle with a dropper.

This oil works best if you apply it after a shower or bath. You do not need much, and it spreads and absorbs easily. I have tried this recipe with a few drops of lavender essential oil as well. It really smells nice and can be calming for the skin.

If you have a nut allergy, substitute sunflower oil for the almond oil.

When to Discard: 6 months to a year, depending on shelf life of oils

NIGHTY-NIGHT NECK MASK

Makes 4 ounces

Because the neck does not have the same oil glands as the face and tends to dry out easier, keeping the neck extra hydrated is beneficial. Here is a wonderful neck mask to give your neck a smooth, youthful appearance.

¼ cup shea butter

3 tablespoons castor oil

2 teaspoons beeswax*

1 teaspoon carrot seed oil

7 drops lemon essential oil

Combine all ingredients except the essential oil. Melt in small saucepan over low heat. Once completely melted, remove from heat and add the essential oil. Stir all ingredients until completely combined, and pour into a small container with a lid. Do *not* seal the lid until fully cooled. Let sit for 6 hours or overnight.

Apply to your neck by gently massaging and evenly distributing the mask over the entire neck and décolletage area. Use every evening with nightly routine.

* Use beeswax pastilles, wafers, or beads because they are so much easier to work with and measure than large chunks of beeswax.

When to Discard: about a month

WILD PEPPERMINT BEARD BALM

Makes 1 ounce

1 tablespoon shea butter

1 tablespoon coconut butter

1 tablespoon jojoba oil

½ tablespoon beeswax*

10 drops peppermint essential oil

10 drops grapefruit essential oil

10 drops wild orange essential oil

In small saucepan, combine all ingredients except the essential oils. Melt over low heat, then remove from heat and add the essential oils. Stir thoroughly and pour into small container(s) with a lid. Do *not* seal lid until fully cooled. Let sit for 6 hours or overnight before using.

Apply the balm to your mustache and beard area daily, massaging it into the base of your hair (follicles) and distributing throughout. Use as needed.

* Use beeswax pastilles, wafers, or beads because they are so much easier to work with and measure than large chunks of beeswax.

When to Discard: about 6 months

FRANKINCENSE & LAVENDER
SKIN OINTMENT

Makes 4 ounces

¼ cup raw, unrefined coconut oil

¼ cup jojoba oil

⅛ cup beeswax*

5 drops frankincense essential oil

8 drops lavender essential oil

Warm all ingredients, except the essential oils, on low heat until completely melted. Remove from heat and stir in the essential oils. Let cool completely, about 3 hours. Do *not* seal your container until the ointment has completely cooled. Store in small container(s) with a lid. Use whenever needed.

* Use beeswax pastilles, wafers, or beads because they are so much easier to work with and measure than large chunks of beeswax.

When to Discard: about 6 months

A WORD ON SALVES

One easy way to help repair your skin from an injury is with a salve. Salves are a great way to include herbs and rich oils in your skin-care routine. Many salves use an infused oil, which is when herbs are infused into the oil by either heating them or immersing them in an oil for a long period of time. See page 154 for details about making infusions.

NATURAL SUN PROTECTION

There are two different types of sunrays that are important to understand. These are UVA rays and UVB rays, both of which affect the skin.

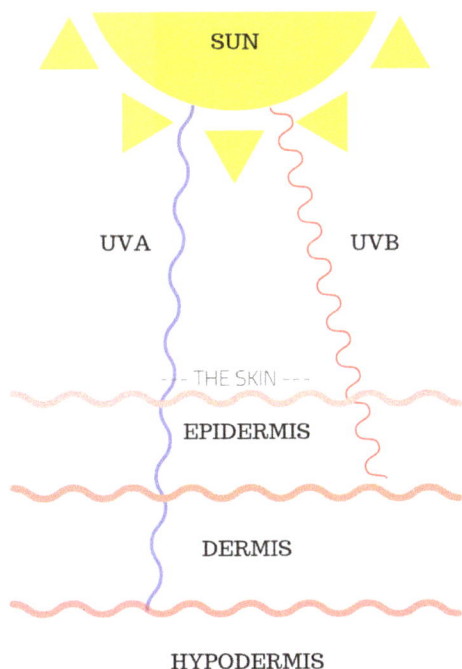

Different rays of the sun and their penetration into the skin

UVA rays can penetrate deep into the skin, causing damage and photo-aging. UVB rays damage the skin's outer layers by causing a sunburn, which can lead to certain skin cancers.

To protect yourself from overexposure to the sun, stay in the shade or wear a wide-brimmed hat and clothing that covers your arms and legs.

The sun is responsible for approximately 80% of aging. That is an incredibly high percentage! As a result of the high percentage of damage the skin may experience, many professionals press the use of sunscreen. However, some sunscreens contain a lot of chemicals and can actually be harmful to your skin.

Some of the most popular supermarket sunscreens contain harmful ingredients such as oxybenzone, octinoxate, homosalate, octisalate and octocrylene, which can cause skin irritation and sensitivity, according to the Environmental Working Group (EWG), a consumer-advocacy organization. These ingredients rank anywhere between a level 3 to a level 8 on EWG's toxicity range, in which level 10 is the worst possible score. (See www. EWG.org/skindeep for more information.)

In my opinion, avoiding overexposure to the sun and wearing a more natural sunscreen is a healthier option.

BETTER BUTTERS
SUN PROTECTION CREAM

*** Making your own sun protection during the summer months is great way to keep your skin nourished and protected in a more natural way. However, one note of caution is that zinc oxide can be harmful to your health if inhaled. Wear rubber gloves and a face mask when working with this mineral compound as it is a very fine powder and can easily get into the lungs. Keep away from children in its powdered form.*

Makes 4 ounces

    1½ tablespoons beeswax*

    3 tablespoons raw, unrefined coconut oil

    2 tablespoons cocoa butter

    ½ tablespoon carrot seed oil (can substitute sunflower or almond oil)

    1 tablespoon zinc oxide powder**

In a pan, melt all ingredients except the zinc oxide on low. Remove from heat and add the zinc oxide. Stir well to make sure the zinc oxide is completely dissolved. Let cool completely, about 8 hours, before pouring into small containers. Because this is an all-natural sun protection lotion, be careful not to leave it anywhere hot as it can melt and shorten the product's shelf life.

Apply liberally any time you will be in the sun. This recipe is considered about a 12% SPF according to the calculation sheet on the next page. However, this formula is not waterproof, so reapply after you get out of the water.

* Use beeswax pastilles, wafers, or beads because they are so much easier to work with and measure than large chunks of beeswax.

When to Discard: about 6 months; refrigeration can prolong shelf life

ZINC OXIDE CALCULATION CHEAT SHEET

Here's how to figure out how much zinc oxide you need to approximate the Sun Protection Factor (SPF) in store-bought products.

If you want to make a low SPF (2% to 5%), then about 5% of your total product volume should be zinc oxide.

If you want to make a moderate SPF (6% to 11%), then about 10% of your total product volume should be zinc oxide.

If you want to make a high SPF (12% to 19%), then 15% of your total product volume should be zinc oxide.

AFTER-SUN REPAIR OIL

Makes 6 ounces

½ cup jojoba oil

⅛ cup carrot seed carrier oil

¼ cup grapeseed oil

7 drops frankincense essential oil

5 drops lavender essential oil

Combine all ingredients and pour into a sealable container that is easy to use, like an amber-colored glass bottle with a dropper.

Apply liberally to skin that has been overexposed to sun. Gently rub in to affected areas as needed.

When to Discard: 6 months to a year, depending on the shelf life of the oils

AFTER-SUN REPAIR SPRAY

Makes 8 ounces

1 cup aloe vera juice

1 teaspoon colloidal silver

10 drops lavender essential oil

5 drops frankincense essential oil

Combine all ingredients into a spray bottle. I prefer amber-colored glass to preserve the colloidal silver.

Shake before each use. Spray thoroughly over irritated skin several times per day.

When to Discard: about 5 months

AFTER-SUN REPAIR OINTMENT

Makes 4 ounces

¼ cup raw, unrefined coconut oil

¼ cup raw honey

1 teaspoon beeswax*

1 full dropper sea buckthorn oil

10 drops lavender essential oil

Over low heat, warm the coconut oil, honey and beeswax until completely melted. Remove from heat and add sea buckthorn oil and lavender essential oil. Let cool completely, about 3 hours. Do *not* seal your container until the ointment has completely cooled. Store in a small container(s) with a lid.

Gently apply to sunburned skin as needed.

* Use beeswax pastilles, wafers, or beads because they are so much easier to work with and measure than large chunks of beeswax.

When to Discard: about a month

COOLING-MINT REPAIR GEL

Makes 2 ounces

¼ cup aloe vera gel

2 tablespoons raw, unrefined coconut oil

1 teaspoon colloidal silver

½ teaspoon glycerin

5 drops tea tree essential oil

3 drops peppermint essential oil

2 drops sage essential oil

Combine all ingredients in a container with a lid. I prefer amber-colored glass to preserve the colloidal silver. Stir before each use.

Apply to irritated, burned, or chapped skin several times per day.

When to Discard: about a month

CHAPTER 13

Bath & Body Care:

FROM MASSAGE OIL TO DEODORANT

B ath and body products are my favorite creations because they always make great gifts. These products—which range from lotions and bath powders to body butters—can be tailored to a loved one's tastes by using their favorite scent and color. Sweet-smelling bath salts or fizzing bath bombs wrapped in delicate paper or with the recipient's favorite dried flower can make such meaningful and heartfelt gifts.

FOOT SOAKS

In this chapter you will find recipes for luxury bath and body products, intended for self-care. Foot soaks are a great way to bring relaxation to the body and make wonderful self-care gifts for others or for spa parties. Foot soaks, which contain salts and minerals, offer instant relaxation. Many who use mineral salts for detox baths report relief from aches and pains, reduced inflammation, improved circulation and relief from a variety of ailments. Epsom and Himalayan salts have been used for centuries for different health remedies.

The three main ingredients I like to use in my foot soaks and bath treatments are Epsom salts, magnesium flakes, and Himalayan salts. I like this combination as I believe these ingredients all offer different benefits.

Magnesium deficiency in the body can often lead to foot and leg cramps. These muscle spasms can be annoying and painful. A refreshing, detoxifying foot bath allows for magnesium absorption through the skin. Topical magnesium has personally helped my own aches and pains, and I often use detoxifying bath salts for sore muscles or if I am fighting a cold.

Give the refreshing foot detox, in the next section, a try. You can also try adding your own favorite essential oil blends.

MAGNESIUM-PACKED FOOT DETOX

Makes 16 ounces

This recipe is great for a spa party—or just for an afternoon of personal pampering.

> 1 cup Epsom salts
>
> ¼ cup magnesium flakes
>
> ¼ cup Himalayan salt
>
> 8 drops peppermint essential oil
>
> 6 drops orange essential oil
>
> 5 drops eucalyptus essential oil

In a large bowl, combine Epsom and Himalayan salts with the essential oils. Mix well, then stir in the magnesium flakes, and pour into 2 to 8 ounce containers with lids.

Pour about 6 cups of warm water into a basin large enough for your feet. Add 2 or 3 tablespoons of the foot detox mix into the water and let it dissolve. Relax and soak your feet for about 10 minutes.

You can also add stones to the bottom of the basin and/or petals to float on top the water. It is fun to be creative with different recipes. I love the peppermint essential oil mixture above because it leaves my feet a little tingly. You will want to use your detox salts within a week or so because the magnesium flakes have a tendency to dissolve when mixed with essential oils.

When to Discard: about a week

REFRESHING PEPPERMINT BATH SALTS

Makes 8 ounces

Bathing in hot water can cause your body to sweat out toxins, giving you another added benefit to taking a detoxifying salt bath. Be sure to drink extra water, as sweating out toxins can dehydrate the body. Try out a spa water for some different hydration options, as listed in Chapter 18.

½ cup Epsom salts

½ cup sea salt

1 teaspoon baking soda

1 teaspoon jojoba oil

10 drops peppermint essential oil

Combine all ingredients in a bowl and transfer to a pourable plastic container with a lid. Add approximately 1 to 2 tablespoons of bath salts to warm bathwater.

When to Discard: about 6 months

GENTLE LAVENDER BATH SALTS FOR KIDS

Makes 6 ounces

Occasionally, when the kids were not feeling well, I put some bath salts into the tub. I found that it made them feel better and helped them sleep. Many bath products for children can be full of unwanted ingredients, which are not beneficial when they are fighting colds. Himalayan salts and Epsom salts also help little ones relax in the warm tub.

¼ cup pink Himalayan salt

½ cup Epsom salts

½ tablespoon sunflower oil

10 drops lavender essential oil

Mix all ingredients together in a bowl. Store in a container with a lid.

Add about 1 tablespoon of bath salt mixture to the bathtub. (I do not recommend this for children under one year of age because essential oils can be too strong for infants.)

When to Discard: about 4 months

FIZZING BATH TRUFFLES

Makes 8 to 10 small truffles

Have you ever tried to make your own bath bombs only to have them crumble on you, dry out your skin, or turn out not quite right? I have tried many different bath bomb recipes and experienced all these unpleasant results. The fizzing bath truffle is different than most recipes and is my absolute favorite.

Soothing cocoa butter helps hydrate your skin while the Himalayan salt provides healing benefits for the body. This recipe, which is a little more gentle on the skin than the typical bath bomb recipes you will find online, creates a luxurious bath experience with just the right ingredients to soften the skin.

   2½ tablespoons cocoa-butter wafers

   ½ cup baking soda

   1 tablespoon Himalayan salt

   3 tablespoons citric acid (powder)

   10 drops ylang ylang essential oil

In a small saucepan, warm the cocoa butter on low heat. As soon as it is completely melted, remove from heat and add baking soda, Himalayan salt, and the citric acid powder. Mix quickly, then add the essential oils. Mix again and press into a silicone-type mold made for ice cubes or candies. The mixture should be a thick, paste-like consistency. Put it in the refrigerator and let cool it for about 2 hours. Pop out your bath truffles and store in a cool, dry place.

Place one or two bath truffles into a warm bath and watch them bubble away.

When to Discard: about 4 months

MOISTURIZING OAT CLEANSING BAR

Makes 18 ounces

The Moisturizing Oat Cleansing Bar can feel gummy or sticky when you first use it, but after you rinse off, your skin feels amazing. I have to admit, this can take a little getting used to because it is not your typical bar of soap. However, once you start using these bars, you will not want to stop. They are perfect for travel because you can make them small enough for a couple of uses (or even one use). They cleanse and moisturize at the same time, and they leave your skin feeling soft and smooth without the need to apply lotion after you shower.

1 cup oat flour	1 tablespoon olive oil
¼ cup cocoa butter wafers	½ cup Himalayan salt
¼ cup shea butter	1 tablespoon kaolin clay powder
2 tablespoons beeswax pastilles*	15 drops wild orange essential oil (optional)

On low heat, warm cocoa butter, shea butter, beeswax, and olive oil until melted. Remove from heat. Combine all other ingredients and mix well. Pour into small silicone molds. I use small square or floral-shaped molds, and I prefer molds about 1.5 inches across, around the size of a golf ball. Put in the refrigerator for several hours to let cool completely. Once the bars have hardened, pop them out of the silicone molds and let them continue to set up at room temperature for a couple more hours. For firmer bars, increase the beeswax by another tablespoon.

Use in the bath or shower in place of soap.

* Use beeswax pastilles, wafers, or beads because they are so much easier to work with and measure than large chunks of beeswax.

When to Discard: about 2 months, depending on shelf life of oils

COCONUT-ALMOND CLEANSING MILK

This is one of my favorite body wash recipes. It smells so pretty and leaves the skin soft and clean. It is even gentle enough to use on the face.

Makes 5 ounces

¼ cup almond castile soap

2 tablespoons condensed milk

¼ cup raw, unrefined coconut oil

½ teaspoon almond extract

Heat the coconut oil on low, just enough to melt, and remove from heat. Add condensed milk and remaining ingredients. Stir well and let completely cool. Pour into a container with a pump. (You can double this recipe for larger batch.)

Use all over your body in the shower as needed.

When to Discard: about 2 months

MINT-MOLASSES BODY WASH

Makes 5 ounces

¼ cup peppermint castile soap

½ teaspoon peppermint extract (or peppermint flavor)

¼ cup raw, unrefined coconut oil

1 tablespoon molasses

4-5 drops eucalyptus essential oil* (optional)

Heat coconut oil on low, just enough to melt, and remove from heat. Add molasses and remaining ingredients. Stir well and let completely cool. Pour into a container with a pump. Use all over body in the shower as needed. Can double recipe for larger batch.

* Omit eucalyptus essential oil if you are using this body wash on young children or if you have sensitive skin.

When to Discard: about 1 month

BUBBLING ORANGE BATH POWDER

Makes 8 ounces

¾ cup baking soda

¼ cup pink Himalayan salt

¼ cup citric acid (powder)

1 tablespoon goat milk powder or regular dehydrated milk powder

10 drops wild orange essential oil

Combine all ingredients. Smash the essential oils into the powdered mixture to spread as evenly as possible. Store in a pretty glass jar with a lid.

Pour a couple of tablespoons at a time into your bathwater until you have the desired amount.

When to Discard: about 3 months

CLEOPATRA'S MILK & HONEY BATH SOAK

Makes 16 ounces

Bathing in milk and honey was one of Egyptian queen Cleopatra's private rituals. Milk and honey soften the skin, exfoliate naturally, and have a fresh and sweet scent. You can actually make your own milk bath with the following recipe:

2 cups whole milk

½ cup honey

5–8 drops frankincense essential oil*

Warm milk and honey on low heat until the honey is dissolved. Remove from stove and add frankincense essential oil.

Pour the mixture into extra warm bathwater. Soak in the tub and relax.

* I love frankincense oil because it is calming and great for the skin. However, lavender, myrrh, and/or geranium are nice as well.

When to Discard: Use right away, do not store

LAVENDER BODY BUTTER

Makes 12 ounces

This recipe has a consistency like a salve, and it is much easier to make than "whipped" body butter recipes. Lavender Body Butter is one of my favorite recipes because it helps cracked hands and feet or extremely dry skin—especially in winter months! I also use this body butter on eczema breakouts and have had great results.

¼ cup shea butter

½ cup grapeseed oil

¼ cup almond oil*

1 tablespoon rosehip seed oil

2 tablespoons beeswax**

1 teaspoon vitamin E

¼ teaspoon xanthan gum

⅛ teaspoon sea buckthorn oil (optional)

10 drops lavender essential oil

7 drops ylang ylang essential oil (optional)

On low heat, warm all ingredients except xanthan gum and essential oils until completely melted. Let the mixture cool for a few minutes, then stir in xanthan gum. Once xanthan gum is completely dissolved, add in essential oils. Pour into desired containers. Let cool completely, about 3 hours. Do not seal your container until it has completely cooled.

Apply day and night as needed for dry skin. Also, this body butter is a great gift since it makes a larger batch. It smells amazing and is great for the skin!

If you have a nut allergy, substitute sunflower oil or another oil of your choice.

***Use beeswax pastilles, wafers, or beads because they are so much easier to work with and measure than large chunks of beeswax.*

When to Discard: about 2 months

CINNAMON-ALOE BODY MOISTURIZER

Makes 5 ounces

Some body butters can be a little too heavy or greasy on the skin, which makes an aloe moisturizer a perfect alternative. This cinnamon-scented, light moisturizer will leave your skin feeling soft and refreshed.

½ cup aloe vera gel

2 teaspoons castor oil

1/2 teaspoon jojoba oil

¼ teaspoon cinnamon powder

2 drops cinnamon food grade flavor or extract (optional)

Combine all ingredients with a whisk to evenly distribute the cinnamon. Transfer to a pump bottle and shake well.

Apply as needed, rubbing the moisturizer into your skin until it is absorbed. Gently shake before each use if necessary.

When to Discard: about a month

LEMON-PEPPERMINT FOOT CREAM

Makes 8 ounces

I like to keep my feet soft all year round so I began using different foot creams. The essential oils in this blend provide a bit of a cooling effect and can help smooth out calluses. I apply this foot cream only at night after I am in bed because it can be a bit greasy. In the morning your feet will be nice and soft.

¼ cup shea butter

½ cup grapeseed oil

¼ cup almond oil

2 tablespoon beeswax*

1 tablespoon glycerin

¼ teaspoon xanthan gum

12 drops peppermint essential oil

10 drops lemon essential oil

8 drops tea tree essential oil

Combine the shea butter with the beeswax in a small saucepan and melt over low heat. Remove from heat and add all other ingredients except xanthan gum and essential oils. Stir together, then add in the xanthan gum and essential oils.

Whip together with a handheld mixer, removing as many lumps as possible. The mixture should be a creamy, light yellow color. Pour into desired container and let cool for at least 4 hours. I like to let mine sit overnight. Do *not* seal your container until it has completely cooled. This product may begin to separate after several weeks.

* Use beeswax pastilles, wafers, or beads because they are so much easier to work with and measure than large chunks of beeswax.

When to Discard: about a month

WHAT IS XANTHAN GUM?

Xanthan gum (also known as *Xanthomonas campestris*) is a type of sugar or polysaccharide, that is made from bacteria. When these bacteria are fed glucose, they secrete a sticky substance that scientists have figured out how to dry and make into powder form. I always try to get a high-quality xanthan gum to avoid too many chemicals being used in this process.

Xanthan gum is used mostly in baking as an all-purpose thickener. It is a great substitute in gluten-free recipes as it acts as a binder. The same is true for skin-care products. It is a more natural way to get your products to thicken and bind together.

CALMING "CALAMINE" LOTION

My kids always ask me to make this recipe at the beginning of summer as it instantly calms the itch of pesky mosquito bites. This formulation can also be applied as an overnight zit cream for pimples! It will calm an irritated pimple for a quicker recovery.

Makes 4 ounces

¼ cup zinc oxide (powder)*

4 teaspoons pink kaolin clay

4 teaspoons baking soda

¼ cup aloe vera

½ teaspoon glycerin

4 drops tea tree essential oil

Whisk all ingredients in a bowl until completely smooth. Put into a container with a lid.

Apply to irritated skin or mosquito/bug bites as needed.

* Zinc-oxide powder can be harmful to your health if inhaled. Wear rubber gloves and a face mask when working with this product. Keep away from children in its original, powdered form.

Caution: Be careful, as this dried lotion can rub off on your pillow and be a bit messy if you are using it in a lot of areas on your face.

When to Discard: about a week (can keep in refrigerator to prolong use)

WARM VANILLA MASSAGE OIL

Makes 8 ounces

A romantic and inexpensive gift you can make for a loved one is a warming massage oil. Light and sweet smelling, it is beneficial for sore muscles and promotes relaxation. The ingredients are simple but intentional. Chili peppers contain capsaicin, which help desensitize pain receptors. Crushed red pepper, when infused with oil, will give a tingle or warming sensation vs. a hot sensation. However, it will still ease tense muscles and offer relief. See more about chili pepper benefits in the Glossary of Skin-Friendly Ingredients.

> 1 cup fractionated coconut oil
>
> 1 teaspoon ginger, dried and crushed
>
> 1 teaspoon dried red chili pepper, crushed
>
> ½ vanilla pod, crushed
>
> 14 drops vanilla essential oil
>
> 4 drops ylang ylang essential oil

Combine coconut oil, ginger, red pepper, and vanilla pod. Heat on low for several minutes until oil becomes very hot. (For a more intense oil, try making an infusion. See the infusion instructions on page 154.) Do *not* bring to a boil. Remove from heat and let cool for several hours. Strain and transfer oil to an 8-ounce container. Use a cheesecloth in your funnel to strain out the solid ingredients.

Your oil will be a rich, golden color with flecks of vanilla. (Beautiful!) Add the essential oils to your container and shake gently to distribute. The massage oil is now ready.

Apply liberally to the skin and massage into sore muscles. Avoid touching sensitive areas such as your eyes—even after use—because this recipe contains chili peppers. Though this recipe smells good enough to eat, I don't recommend it unless you omit the essential oils.

When to Discard: about 6 months

CALMING ROSEMARY MASSAGE OIL

Makes 12 ounces

1 cup grapeseed oil

½ cup fractionated
coconut oil

15 drops rosemary essential oil

5 drops tea tree essential oil

Combine all ingredients. Store in a container with a pump.

Use this massage oil when you need to relax from stress or exhaustion.

When to Discard: about a year, depending on shelf life of oils

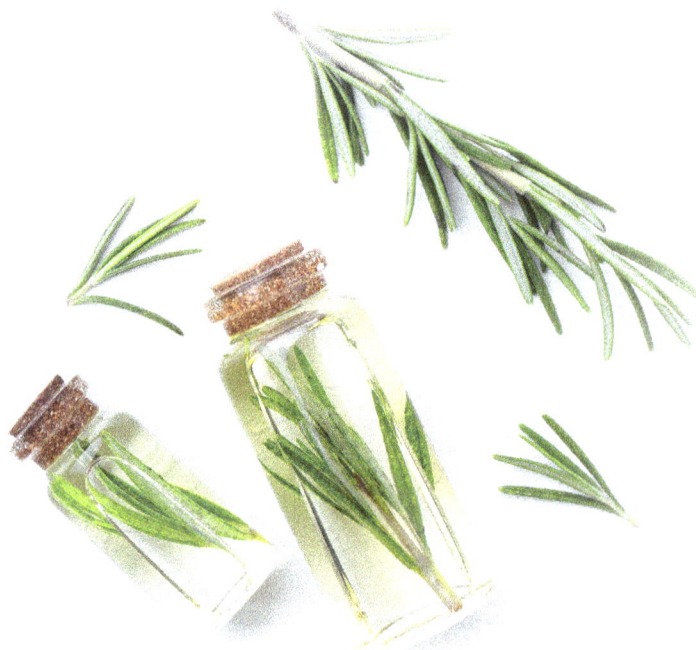

THE QUEST FOR NATURAL DEODORANT

When it comes to deodorant, there are more than enough to choose from, but which one is right for you? I myself have tried dozens of common brands, but once I learned about the harmful chemicals in most deodorants, I switched to a natural brand. Sadly, it did not work—at all. So I switched to another natural one, and another. I have to be honest, they just did *not* work for me. So I tried a few DIY recipes at home to see if they were any better. Thankfully, after a bit of trial and error, I found one that really works! And I know exactly what is in it.

COMMON DEODORANT INGREDIENTS

- Triclosan

- Aluminum (aluminum chlorohydrate, aluminum zirconium tetra-chlorohydrex or any aluminum compounds)

- Polyethylene glycol (PEG), steareth, propylene glycol

- Parabens (methyl, ethyl, propyl, benzyl, and butyl)

- Phthalates

- Fragrance

- Butylated hydroxytoluene (BHT), butylated hydroxyanisole (BHA)

- Talc

Many deodorant ingredients can be harmful to your health. Since this is a product that is applied to the skin (sometimes more than once a day) and left on all day instead of rinsed off, it is important that the ingredients are not harmful to your overall health. Deodorant roll-ons are often more of a water consistency and easily absorbed into the skin. I encourage you to do your own research on ingredients, but my findings are in the product-ingredient reference that starts on page 218. Instead of being at the mercy of a big industry and not knowing exactly what is in your deodorant, just make your own.

COCONUT DEODORANT STICK

Many essential oils are effective deodorizers that help minimize odor and kill bacteria, such as tea tree, ylang ylang, orange, and lemon. Ylang ylang and tea tree are also gentle on the skin, making them a nice combination for a gentle deodorant.

Makes 3 sticks

6 tablespoons raw, organic coconut oil

½ cup + 1 tablespoon pure baking soda

½ cup pure arrowroot (starch/flour)

1 ½ tablespoons organic beeswax*

10–15 drops essential oils**

Combine all ingredients in a pot and heat on low heat until everything is mixed well and melted. Do not overheat. Let cool slightly in pan, then pour into deodorant containers. Put containers in the refrigerator for about 4 hours or let sit overnight before using. Buy empty deodorant containers off Amazon or sanitize used-up containers that you have.

Use beeswax pastilles, wafers, or beads because they are so much easier to work with and measure than large chunks of beeswax.

** *Choose from one of these antiseptic essential oils: tea tree, ylang ylang, orange, and lemon.*

When to Discard: about 3 months

CHAPTER 14

Hair Care for

THE WHOLE FAMILY

Because many of us are concerned about hair growth and hair care, I thought the topic should have its own section. By being immersed in the skin-care world, I have learned a great deal about hair as well as skin. Hair is a chain of proteins that grow from follicles found in the dermis. We have millions of small, tubular glands all over our skin that produce watery fluids that cool the body by evaporation.

The glands at the opening of the hair produce an oil that lubricates the hair and skin. It is quite a complicated dynamic. Really, having good hair-care products is just as important as good skin-care products. When I began replacing all of my family's body products, I was appalled to learn what was in our hair-care products as well, especially the ones for children.

My daughter's hair is very fine and tangles easily. As a result, I use a detangler on her hair every morning. Some of the children's hair products smell nice and have fun colors and pictures on the bottle, so they seem like such innocent products. However, after looking at the ingredients of standard children's hair detanglers, I could no longer use them.

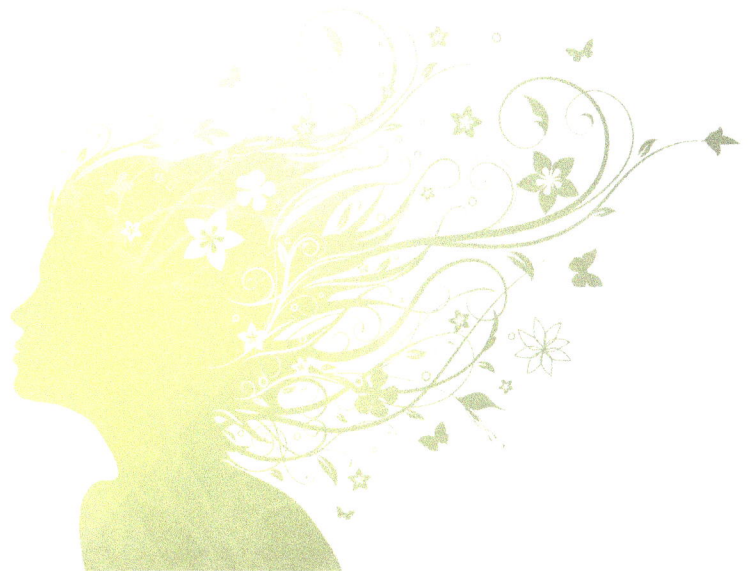

COMMON INGREDIENTS IN HAIR DETANGLERS

Propylene glycol

Polysorbate 20

Fragrance (parfum)

Amodimethicone

DMDM hydantoin

Cetrimonium chloride

Tetrasodium polyquaternium-10

Citric acid

Butylene glycol

Iodopropynyl butylcarbamate

Methylchloroisothiazolinone/ methylisothiazolinone

Many of these I consider to be toxic, but since a detangler really made our mornings easier, I was determined to find an alternative that worked.

Another awesome reason to make your own hair-detangling spray is that you can add ingredients that repel lice and bugs. As parents, many of us have experienced first hand the stress of a lice outbreak at school. It is common to get warnings from teachers about not letting children share coats or backpacks, a practice that can spread infestation. Just the word "lice" freaks many of us out. Using hair care ingredients like thyme, peppermint, and sage can actually reduce a child's risk of getting these tiny bugs in their hair.

PROTECTIVE HERBAL HAIR DETANGLER

Makes 8 ounces

This recipe smells amazing! I reduced the amount of aloe vera in the recipe because fine hair tends to get greasy. However, if you need more moisture in your detangler, add a second tablespoon of aloe vera to your mix. I use this combination on everyone's hair, even my own. Thyme and peppermint not only repel lice, but are also known to stimulate hair growth, which is another added bonus.

¾ cup filtered water

¼ cup vodka*

1 tablespoon pure aloe vera juice

10 drops thyme essential oil

10 drops sage essential oil

10 drops rosemary essential oil

10 drops peppermint essential oil

5 drops cinnamon bark (not cassia) essential oil

Pour all ingredients into a metal or glass spray bottle. Shake before each use.

Just a few spritzes of this detangler are needed on your hair. A little goes a long way.

Do not be alarmed that there is vodka in your recipe. Vodka is considered a grain alcohol, and I prefer it over rubbing alcohol; however you can use witch hazel as a substitute.

When to Discard: about three months

THE BENEFITS OF DRY SHAMPOO

Using a dry shampoo can have multiple purposes. First, it saves money as the ingredients are inexpensive. Additionally, some of the ingredients have added benefits. For example, rosemary stimulates hair growth and can be used to prevent premature graying and dandruff. It may also help dry or itchy scalp.

Another ingredient I love is cinnamon, which can also stimulate your scalp. It may tingle a bit, however it is believed that the sensation is actually the stimulating of hair follicles that helps with hair growth. The natural scent is a perfect asset for a hair powder.

FRESH ROSEMARY HAIR POWDER
(for blonde hair)

Makes 2 ounces

- 2 tablespoons arrowroot powder

- 1 tablespoon baking soda

- ½ teaspoon maca powder

- 5 drops rosemary essential oil

Combine all ingredients in a small container with a lid. I use a small glass jar or disposable condiment container. Carefully blend in the essential oil, making sure it is completely distributed.

Use daily on hair, using a makeup blush brush that is designated only for your dry shampoo. Gently dab the brush into the container and tap it on the lid to eliminate excess. Tap into your hairline and brush it in with your fingertips or a hairbrush.

When to Discard: about 6 months

DARK & PRETTY HAIR POWDER
(for brunette, dark-brown, or black hair)

Makes 4 ounces

This is an amazingly sweet and rich hair powder for dark hair. Grapefruit essential oil can be helpful for healthy hair growth and acts as a wonderful deodorizer.

> 2 tablespoons cocoa powder
>
> 2 tablespoons cornstarch
>
> 2 teaspoons ground cinnamon*
>
> ½ teaspoon cardamom*
>
> 5 drops grapefruit essential oil

Combine all ingredients in a small container with a lid. I use a small glass jar or disposable condiment container.

Use daily on hair, using a makeup blush brush that is designated only for your dry shampoo. Gently dab the brush into the container and tap it on the lid to eliminate excess. Tap into your hairline, and brush it in with your fingertips or a hairbrush.

* Cinnamon and cardamom have been known in some cases to slightly lighten the hair. If you are concerned or notice any change in hair color, omit the spices.

When to Discard: about 6 months

SWEET & SANDY HAIR POWDER
(for light-brown or sandy-blonde hair)

Makes 2 ounces

This combination smells amazing and is also beneficial for hair growth.

> 2 tablespoons cornstarch
>
> 2 tablespoons arrowroot powder
>
> 1 teaspoon ground cinnamon*
>
> ½ teaspoon cardamom*

Combine all ingredients in a small container with a lid. I use a small glass jar or disposable condiment container.

Use daily on hair, using a makeup blush brush that is designated only for your dry shampoo. Gently dab the brush into the container and tap it on the lid to eliminate excess. Tap into your hairline, and brush it in with your fingertips or a hairbrush.

* Cinnamon and cardamom have been known in some cases to slightly lighten the hair. If you are concerned or notice any change in hair color, omit the spices and use 1 teaspoon of cocoa powder instead.

When to Discard: about 6 months

JOJOBA HAIR OIL

Makes 2 ounces

Having an oil on hand to smooth hair follicles and offer a bit of shine can give a person a boost of confidence. This pleasant-smelling hair oil gives a healthy glow to the hair.

> ¼ cup jojoba oil
>
> 1 teaspoon rosehip seed oil
>
> 5 drops rosemary essential oil
>
> 5 drops grapefruit essential oil

Combine all ingredients and pour in a small pump bottle or a glass dropper bottle.

Apply a small amount to hands and evenly distribute through fingertips. Apply to the ends of your hair, and massage the ends to tame frizz. Do not put directly on the scalp.

When to Discard: about 6 months

CLARIFYING APPLE HAIR RINSE

Makes 4 ounces

I love apple cider vinegar (ACV) for its overall health benefits, but I have *never* liked the smell. I do not love using it in products because, the initial scent is unpleasant. Even though this hair rinse does not smell the best when applying it, you cannot beat the benefits! After using an ACV rinse, you will notice your hair is nice and shiny. The vinegar also removes excess oil, acting as a clarifying shampoo. If you can bear the smell, you will love the results!

½ cup apple cider vinegar*

2 drops tea tree essential oil

3 drops rosemary essential oil

Combine ingredients in a container that is easy to take into the shower. After shampooing and rinsing, apply ACV hair rinse. Let sit on hair for a few minutes and then rinse thoroughly. Can apply conditioner, if necessary.

Try making your own apple cider vinegar; see page 197 for instructions. If you make your own cider you can control the taste and strength. Any homemade apple cider vinegar I have made has a much milder, and more enjoyable taste and scent.

When to Discard: Use immediately; do not store.

MEDIUM-HOLD VANILLA HAIRSPRAY

Makes 8 ounces

1 cup filtered water

1 teaspoon vanilla extract

1½ tablespoons pure cane sugar

5 drops vanilla essential oil

2 tablespoons rum or vodka
(40 percent alcohol or 80 proof)

Combine water and sugar in a saucepan and heat until sugar is completely dissolved. Bring to a boil and then remove from heat. Let cool completely. Add remaining ingredients and transfer to a spray bottle. Use on hair as needed. Shake gently before each use.

When to Discard: about 2 months

BACK-TO-THE-SEA SALT SPRAY

Makes 8 ounces

1 cup purified water

1 teaspoon Himalayan salt, finely ground

1 teaspoon Epsom salts

1 teaspoon sea salt

1 teaspoon aloe vera juice

15 drops jasmine essential oil*

Bring water to a boil and remove from heat. Add the salts and stir until completely dissolved. Cool slightly and add aloe vera and the essential oils. Let cool completely, then transfer to a spray bottle.

Use on hair as needed. Shake gently before each use.

* Most jasmine essential oil is blended with another oil. Pure jasmine essential oil is extremely expensive; you would only need one drop versus five of the blended.

When to Discard: about 3 months

WAXING HAIR

I have quite a bit of experience when it comes to waxing hair. Most work days include a brow or facial wax. I waxed my own brows long before I was qualified to do so. When I was learning to wax, I spent a lot of time trying new techniques to see what would be the least painful for a client and leave the best results. I have extremely sensitive skin, so I was easily able to see what techniques and products would be most gentle on others.

Waxing bumps can be a terrible nuisance. When removing hair abruptly from the skin, an imbalance can occur, causing the oil glands to work overtime, and as a result a breakout can occur. It can also be a simple irritation to the wax, the temperature of the wax, or just sensitive skin. Everyone reacts differently. Many times a little irritation can be considered somewhat normal. However, the good news is there are steps you can take to lessen or avoid irritation altogether, even if you have sensitive skin.

BEST WAXING PRACTICES: THE 7 STEPS

Step 1: Remove all makeup and cleanse the skin.

Step 2: Exfoliate the skin.

Step 3: Use a non-irritating wax. Know the type of wax that works best with your skin and whether you have a sensitivity to certain ingredients, such as honey.

Step 4: Keep skin clean after a wax, and avoid touching your skin.

Step 5: Wash your face with a gentle cleanser after you wax. Sometimes a nice warm shower, with the steam, will help replenish moisture and rebalance the skin.

Step 6: Apply a natural moisturizer, oil, or gel, and keep your skin hydrated. If your skin feels itchy, add more moisturizer.

Step 7: Let your clean skin breathe overnight. Avoid wearing makeup after a wax, and make sure to do your nightly skin-care routine before bed.

When following these steps, you greatly reduce the possibility of having a reaction to waxing. I highly recommend that you hire a professional to wax your eyebrows and facial area. However, if you choose to wax on your own, there are a few *very* important things you should know.

First, the wax should never be burning-lava hot. If you are able to find a hard wax or one that does not need to be heated to high temperatures, that would be ideal. Second, if you are using a wax that requires strips to be applied and pulled off, be sure to press strips firmly to the skin before removing. Wax and strips should always be applied in the direction of hair growth, then should be removed the in the opposite direction. The skin should always be pulled tight before removing wax to avoid tearing the skin. Be sure to follow the guidelines above when doing your own waxing.

HOW TO SHAPE YOUR EYEBROWS

Unfortunately, many of us are not taught that we need to keep our eyebrows tidy. Eyebrows frame your eyes and make such a difference when they are maintained. When shaped well they can really bring out the color and shape of your eyes and accentuate your facial features. Here is an easy guide on how to shape them:

1. Inside Edge: Line up your tear duct with the beginning of your brow by using a pencil and setting it at the edge of the nose. Where your pencil touches your brow is usually a good indication of where your eyebrow should begin.

2. The Arch: To find the arch, set the pencil at the edge of the nose while looking directly ahead. Set the pencil directly over the iris of the eye. That is where your arch most likely should occur.

3. The Outside Edge: Angle a pencil from the side of the nose to the outside corner of your eye to see where the brow should end.

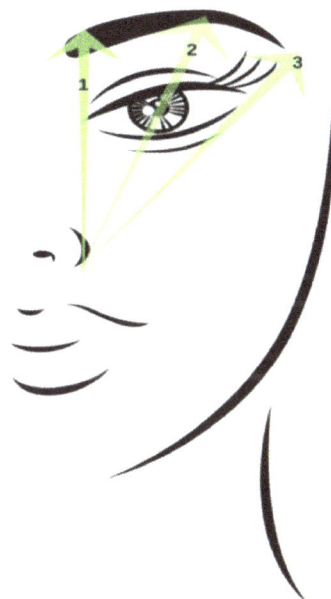

Sometimes there are a few hairs remaining after a wax, so you may need to tweeze those stragglers. Some prefer tweezing over waxing. In either case, there are a few things to know about yanking those little hairs. When tweezing, it is important to always pull the hair out in the same direction it is lying, never "against the grain." Pulling against the grain can cause the hair to break instead of coming out clean. It helps to tweeze the hairs when the skin is pulled somewhat tight. After a hot shower, the pores open up and it is a little easier to tweeze. Also using a bit of witch hazel on a cotton ball before and after tweezing acts as an astringent and can calm and balance the skin.

One last step to complete the perfect brow is to trim. For those longer hairs, simply brush them all up with an eyebrow brush and trim them with a grooming scissors to fit in with the brow line. If the longer hair is much coarser and will not blend well with the others, yank it. But if you can get it to blend, just trim it.

Keeping your brows tidy can be extremely attractive. Do not let the brows form into one—ever—regardless of gender. Unibrows are not flattering. Another thing to remember about eyebrows is that they are sisters (or brothers) *not* twins. There will always be that one eyebrow that is a little different from the other because we are not symmetrical.

Additionally, we all have our own unique shape. In the illustration, you will see a few different eyebrow shapes that I see on a daily basis. They are all beautiful! Everyone's face structure is a little bit different. We naturally have our own shape, and each one is unique and perfect. Give a little shaping a try, and see what you think.

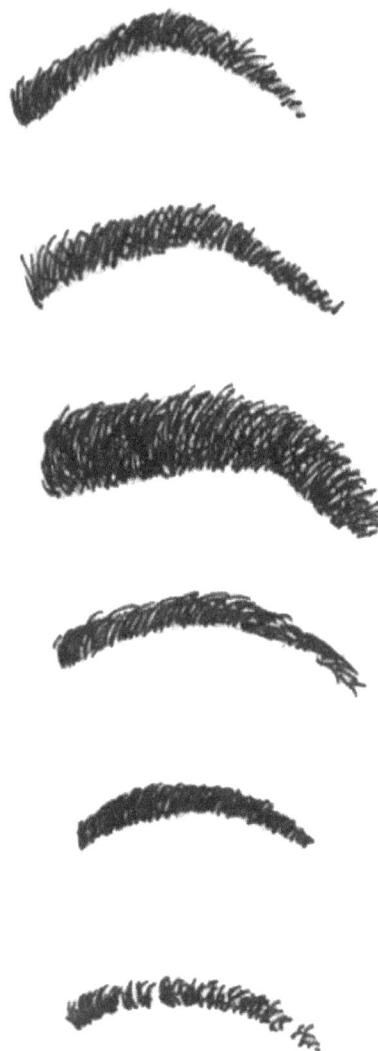

The different shapes of eyebrows

BROW APPEARANCE: MEN VS. WOMEN

The biggest difference between men's eyebrows and women's eyebrows is how defined you make them appear. Follow the same guidelines for a man with less sculpting. However, some men actually prefer their eyebrows a little sharper. This gives a more professional look, which is very popular among businessmen.

A WORD ON SHAVING FOR MEN

There are many ways to get a closer shave and avoid irritation and bumps. A man's facial hair is coarse yet can be more sensitive than expected. Bumps and irritation can be common but not necessary.

Helpful Shaving Tips	
Blades	Use a high-quality razor with a sharp blade, preferably one with multiple blades.
Warm Skin Is Better	Shower before you shave so your skin is warm and pores are open. Or, apply a very warm, wet towel to the skin for several minutes before you shave.
Try a Shaving Brush	A shaving brush made of badger hair retains the most water and gives the best lather.
Gel vs. Cream	Use a shave gel that acts more like a gel and is less like a cream. Shaving gels allow the razor to glide over the skin, causing less irritation.
Direction of Shaving	Go with the grain of the hair in short strokes. Move along one inch at a time.
Be Gentle	Do not press too hard on the skin. If you can feel the blade pressing on your skin, chances are it is causing irritation.
Care for Your Razor Blade	Dry your blade after you shave, and store it in a dry place as this will keep the blade sharp and help it last longer.
Quality Is Better	Higher quality brushes and razors can make all the difference. Try a high-quality razor, one which you are only replacing the blades.

CHAPTER 15

The Power of Aromatherapy

AND NATURAL PERFUMES

Aromatherapy is the use of aromatic plant extracts and essential oils in a massage, bath, or perfume. It can also refer to diffusing scent into the air with the intent to calm or affect the body in some way. It is most common to use essential oils for aromatherapy, but that is not the only method. Many seasoned aromatherapists will use fresh herbs or extracts for aromatherapy as well.

Essential oils are made by distilling large amounts of plant and floral material. The extracted oils are very fragrant and highly concentrated. Oils and hydrosols can be used for a variety of different uses, such as a pleasant air freshener, skin-care products, perfume, ailment remedies, and household cleaners. Essential oils most likely have become popular because they are shown to be effective and only a small amount is needed. Hydrosols have similar properties to essential oils but are mostly distilled water with a lighter concentration of infused essential oils.

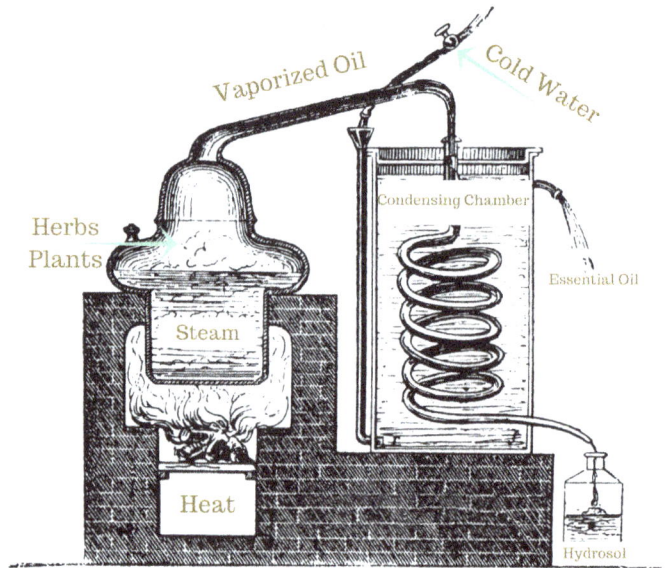

How Essential Oils Are Made

Essential oils are generally made by distilling large quantities of plant material using heat and steam. The plant material releases a vapor, which is condensed and released. The result are highly concentrated oils.

It takes a lot of herbs or plant material to produce essential oils. For example, after distillation of lavender flowers and tops, only about 0.5 to 2 percent of the total yield results in an essential oil. The yield can vary, depending on the type of lavender plants used and the health of the crop. Even more surprising, it takes about sixty whole rosebuds to make one drop of rose essential oil, which is probably why pure rose essential oil is so expensive.

There are approximately 600 drops of essential oil in a one-ounce bottle. The amount of essential oils in personal-care products should be only about 2 percent of the total ingredients. Very little is needed, and as most certified aromatherapists will tell you, do *not* ingest them. Essential oils are of too high a concentration to be taken internally unless under the care of a professional.

WAYS TO USE ESSENTIAL OILS

Topically	Inhalation	Massage	Personal-Care Products
Mix essential oils with your favorite carrier oil and apply directly to the skin. You can do this easily with essential oil rollers.	Apply topical dilution to the palms of your hands and inhale deeply. Or add a few drops to an essential oil diffuser that puts cold steam into the air.	Add a few drops to your body oil or lotion and massage into skin.	Apply to body-care and skin-care products such as serums, bath oils, salts, masks, toners, and scrubs.

MAKING AND USING YOUR OWN ESSENTIAL OIL ROLLERS

It can be fun to play with different essential oil blends. Many oil rollers are used for skin care or aromatherapy. Calming essential oil rollers are very popular right now, as we all tend to have stressful environments or situations that we have to deal with on a daily basis. Stress also makes sleep difficult. Thankfully, essential oil rollers can also be helpful for rest and relaxation. Lavender essential oil has been proven to relieve stress and promote relaxation, as do chamomile, citrus scents, and ylang ylang.

Essential oils should almost always be mixed with a "carrier" oil, which is *not* an essential oil. Typically, carrier oils are mild in nature and easily absorbed into the skin. Some examples of carrier oils are sunflower oil, grapeseed oil, olive oil, and jojoba oil.

When creating your own rollers, make sure not to add too many drops of essential oils, especially if they will be used for children or the elderly. These recommendations are on the safe side. Use a little more or less depending on your sensitivity.

You can purchase essential oil rollers made of glass online at Amazon.com or at your local natural grocery store.

HOW TO MAKE AN ESSENTIAL OIL ROLLER

Essential oil rollers are a handy way to apply essential oils directly to the skin to be absorbed by the body.

1 glass roller bottle (10 ml.)

A carrier oil of your choice*

Essential oil or oils

Simply fill your glass essential oil roller with a carrier oil, leaving a little room at the top of the roller. Apply the desired amount of essential oil drops. Seal with the roller cap and lid.

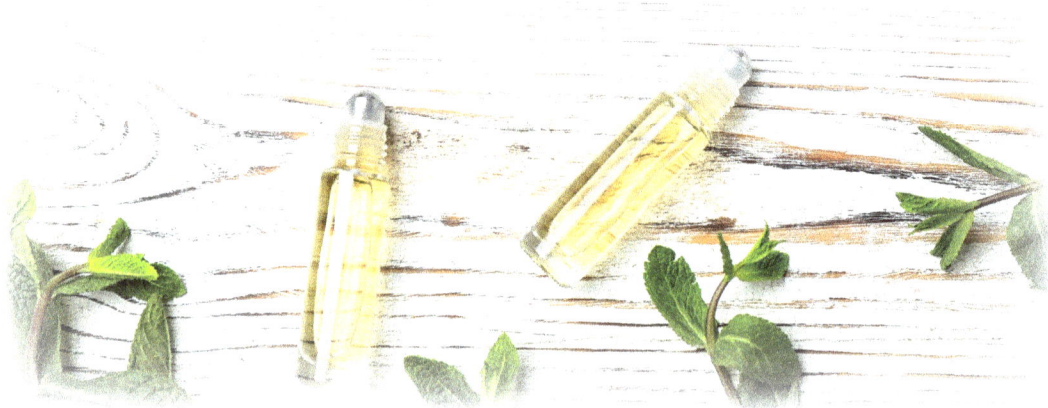

Suggested Guidelines for Essential Oil Rollers	
Children and elderly people	2 drops of each essential oil per 10 ml. (no more than two different essential oils per roller)
Healthy adults	4 drops of each essential oil per 10 ml. (no more than three different essential oils per roller)
Therapeutic dose (for healthy adults only)	6 drops of each essential oil per 10 ml. (no more than three different essential oils per roller)

TIPS FOR USING ESSENTIAL OILS

Where to Apply: The most popular places to apply essential oil rollers are the wrists, temples, and bottoms of the feet.

How Often to Use: Apply one to two times per day, or as needed. Many essential oils are applied at bedtime for restful sleep.

Buying Essential Oils: I prefer to use organic essential oils. These can be purchased at a variety of different places, including Mountain Rose Herbs (www.MountainRoseHerbs.com). When buying essential oils and other ingredients for your beauty products, I strongly encourage you to do your research on the company and the quality of the products being purchased.

A Few of My Favorite Essential Oils and Their Properties	
Clary sage	Stress reducer, antibacterial, balances the body
Eucalyptus	Antiviral and decongestant, great for colds and fevers. Eucalyptus can irritate the skin.
Frankincense	Antibacterial, healing, great for wounds and colds
Grapefruit	Antiseptic, antibacterial, antimicrobial, uplifting scent
Lavender	Antiseptic, antimicrobial, great for sunburns, immune system, and calming anxiety
Lemon	Antiseptic, brightening and bactericidal
Peppermint	Decongestant, antiviral, antiseptic, and expectorant. Great for colds.
Rose	Anti-inflammatory, calms and nourishes the skin
Rosemary	Antiseptic, deep cleansing and antimicrobial
Tea tree (Melaleuca)	Bactericidal, anti-infection. Calms bug bites, cuts and scrapes.
Wild orange	Antiseptic, smells amazing, brightening
Vanilla	Reduces inflammation, reduces stress, antioxidant properties, aromatherapy
Ylang ylang	Gives a person a sense of calm and relaxation, soothes the nerves.

THE POWER OF FRANKINCENSE

Frankincense is obtained from the trees of the genus Boswellia and is also known as olibanum. Its name originally meant "pure or high-quality incense." The essential oil is extracted through steam distillation from the gum resin from the Boswellia tree or shrub, which grows wild throughout northeastern Africa, especially Somalia.

Most of us are familiar with frankincense from the Biblical story of the three Wise Men who brought gifts to the newborn King, Jesus, as described in Matthew 2:11. The fact that frankincense was a gift for such an important occasion shows its true significance. In ancient times, the resin was burned in temples and was considered sacred. Even before we had evidence of its true value, frankincense was highly regarded. This valuable resin was found in ancient Egyptian tombs dating back to 3000 BC. Some traditional churches still use frankincense to this day.

In 2013, Leicester University researchers found that AKBA (acetyl-11-keto-beta-boswellic acid), a chemical compound in the resin, has cancer-killing properties and the potential to destroy ovarian cancer cells. Unfortunately, in our current society, many of us lean toward man-made, synthetic products for healing. Thankfully, frankincense is readily available for use.

POWERFUL FRANKINCENSE ESSENTIAL OIL ROLLER

Makes 10 milliliters

A carrier oil, such as sunflower oil

5–10 drops of frankincense essential oil

Fill a glass essential oil roller (10 ml. size) with a carrier oil, leaving a little room at the top of the roller. Add the frankincense. Secure the cap and lid. Gently shake.

Apply as needed around cuts and scrapes, but never on an open wound. Roll the essential oil roller onto wrists, feet, back of the neck, or forehead for relief from a cold.

Caution: This amazing essential oil can cause vivid dreams in some individuals. If you have trouble sleeping or do not like this side effect, do not use it at bedtime.

When to Discard: depending on carrier oil, can last up to 2 years

PERFUME: USING GOOD SCENTS

I have always loved perfume; however, after learning that there are very loose regulations on these beautiful-smelling products, I began looking for more natural solutions. The majority of chemicals in most commercial fragrances are synthetic compounds derived from petroleum and natural gas, known as petrochemicals. These fragrances are allowed to be 100 percent synthetic. Forget smelling like flowers! It is just chemicals. In addition, perfume manufacturers are allowed to withhold ingredients to protect trade secrets, so who knows what is actually lurking in their fragrances?

Because ingredients are not required to be disclosed on labels, perfumes can end up being a chemical cocktail that are potentially toxic to overall health. Not only are we putting these ingredients directly on our skin but we also breathe them in, as they are normally in a spritz bottle. For that reason, I have been playing with different essential oil combinations. Thankfully, making your own perfume is really fun as it gives you the ability to be creative and tailor the scent to exactly what you want.

The formula I like to use is a three-step process. The base is always a grain alcohol, and I use vodka or rum. I mainly prefer vodka because it does not carry a scent with it. Instead it allows the scent of the essential oils to really be brought out. Rum, on the other hand, has a pleasing sweet scent, which allows the essential oils to have an even sweeter smell to them.

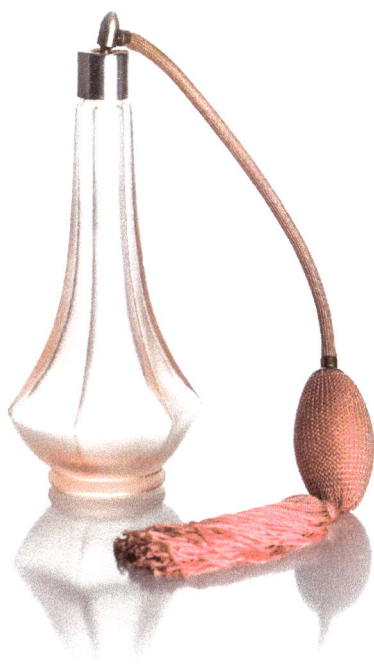

HOW TO MAKE YOUR OWN PERFUME

Step 1: Pour your grain alcohol into a 2 ounce spritz container made of dark glass. Leave about a half-inch space toward the top of the bottle.

Step 2: Add 1/2 teaspoon of either almond, vanilla, or orange extract (or an extract that you prefer) to the alcohol. I like almond extract best.

Step 3: Add three different essential oils. Why three? It is *generally* my rule of thumb. I have found that three scents mixed together always produce the most beautiful combination. Not only that, but three keeps it simple. That being said, I do have a few combinations with more essential oils, but initially I start with three.

Always include at least one strong essential oil scent in combinations to "carry" the scent. For a 2 ounce bottle of perfume you will use a total of about 50 to 75 drops of essential oil. I know that sounds like a large amount of essential oil, but you will only be using a few sprays at a time. A good way to decide whether or not you will like a perfume combination is to test it first. Add a few drops of each essential oil you select to about a teaspoon of carrier oil. This will allow you to try it out before you use a large amount of essential oil for a perfume.

Here's a guide for selecting scents for your favorite natural perfume:

Strong Essential Oils (choose 1)	Blending Essential Oils (choose 2)
Cedarwood	Bergamot
Cinnamon or Cassia	Chamomile
Clove	Clary sage
Frankincense	Grapefruit
Geranium	Lavender
Lemongrass	Lemon
Myrrh	Peppermint
Neroli	Rose
Sandalwood	Rosemary
Vetiver	Vanilla
Ylang ylang	Wild Orange or Orange

Using healing essential oils as your perfume can be so much healthier than what is offered in department stores. The lists of essential oils above are just suggestions. Certain oils that you absolutely love may not be listed. Do not be afraid to give them a try. Once you find a combination that you love, you will always have that recipe for the future. Or, try the blends in the recipes below.

ORANGE-BLOSSOM PERFUME SPRAY

Makes 2 ounces

Vodka or rum (40% alcohol or 80 proof)

20 drops rose essential oil blend (for pure rose use only 5 drops)*

10 drops jasmine essential oil

20 drops orange essential oil

10 drops vanilla essential oil

¼ teaspoon orange extract

Pour grain alcohol into a 2 ounce spritz container made of dark glass. Be sure to leave half an inch of space at the top. Add essential oils and orange extract.

Shake before each use, then spray all over your body whenever needed.

Most rose essential oil is blended with another oil. Pure rose essential oil is extremely expensive and you would need only one drop for every four of the blended.

When to Discard: about a year

SANDY-CITRUS PERFUME SPRAY

Makes 2 ounces

Vodka or rum (40% alcohol or 80 proof)

½ teaspoon almond extract

25 drops frankincense essential oil

25 drops geranium essential oil

20 drops orange essential oil

Pour grain alcohol into a 2 ounce spritz container made of dark glass. Be sure to leave half an inch of space at the top. Add almond extract. Last, add essential oils.

Shake before each use. Spray all over your body whenever needed.

When to Discard: about a year

FRESH-ORANGE LINEN & ROOM SPRAY

Makes 4 ounces

Rum (40% alcohol or 80 proof)

1 teaspoon almond extract

30 drops wild orange essential oil

30 drops tangerine essential oil

10 drops ylang ylang essential oil

Pour grain alcohol into a 2 ounce spritz container made of dark glass. Be sure to leave half an inch of space at the top. Add extract and essential oils.

Shake before each use. Spray generously in the air throughout the room for a sweet, fresh scent.

When to Discard: about a year

SWEET CINNAMON ROOM SPRAY

Makes 4 ounces

Vodka or rum (40% alcohol or 80 proof)

½ teaspoon almond extract

20 drops cinnamon leaf essential oil

20 drops vanilla essential oil blend*

28 drops benzoin essential oil

Pour grain alcohol into a 2 ounce spritz container made of dark glass. Be sure to leave half an inch of space at the top. Add extract and essential oils.

Shake before each use. Spray generously in the air throughout the room for a rich scent of vanilla and cinnamon.

* Most vanilla essential oil is blended with another oil. Pure vanilla essential oil is expensive and you would only need 1 drop for every four of the blended.

When to Discard: about a year

PRETTY SANDALWOOD BODY SPRAY

Makes 4 ounces

Rum (40% alcohol or 80 proof)

1 teaspoon almond extract

30 drops lavender essential oil

30 drops vanilla essential oil blend*

15 drops sandalwood essential oil

Pour grain alcohol into a 2 ounce spritz container made of dark glass. Be sure to leave half an inch of space at the top. Add extract and essential oils.

Shake before each use. Spray generously all over the body for a sweet, musky scent.

* Most vanilla essential oil is blended with another oil. Pure vanilla essential oil is expensive and you would only need 1 drop for every four of the blended.

When to Discard: about a year

SLEEP-WELL PILLOW SPRAY

Makes 2 ounces

Vodka (40% alcohol or 80 proof)

30 drops lavender essential oil

10 drops ylang ylang essential oil

Pour grain alcohol into a 2 ounce spritz container made of dark glass. Be sure to leave half an inch of space at the top. Add essential oils.

Shake before each use. Spray bed pillows whenever needed.

When to Discard: about a year

CHAPTER 16

Preparing Hydrosols, Infusions, and Tinctures

As you may have noticed, some of the recipes in this book refer to ingredients called hydrosols, infusions, and tinctures. This chapter explains what those are, how far in advance you need to prepare them, and how to make them.

Using hydrosols, infusions, and tinctures in skin-care can have many benefits. But trying to understand all the differences and how to make them can be overwhelming. Each method is actually very simple once you get familiar with it. Hydrosols, infusions, and tinctures create a water, oil, or alcohol that is infused with a plant's unique, active constituents.

Hydrosols are pleasant-smelling waters made by distillation of plant materials. These can be used for light, misting sprays for the face and body. The oil infusions, once bottled, can be used directly on the skin or as an ingredient for various hydrating creams and serums as referenced in this book. And finally, tinctures, which are a very popular method of extracting plant material, offer a variety of treatment uses. Tinctures are easy to blend with other water-based liquids and offer a higher concentration of herbal benefits. Below, I go into each method in a little more detail.

HYDROSOLS: DISTILLED FLOWER WATER

Hydrosols are aromatic waters that are created during steam distillation of fresh plants and flowers. They are considered to be gentler and safer to use than essential oils because they are less concentrated. These aromatic waters are a wonderful addition to any skin-care routine.

A great replacement for water in body-care recipes, is a sweet-smelling hydrosol. Some hydrosols can act as a cooling agent, such as a cooling summer facial mist and some can help with balancing oily or dry skin. Hydrosols are a nice toner option as they can be made to be extremely gentle or added into a treatment spray for dry, damaged or sunburned skin. Hydrosols can be used alone or as an ingredient in an herbal treatment spray.

Here are the steps for making a hydrosol:

1. Place washed herbs or flowers into a pot.

2. Add enough water to completely cover the herbs. Bring to a simmer.

3. Place a strainer or other item in the pot so that you can set a bowl on top of it, keeping the bowl from touching the bottom.

4. Place a bowl on the strainer, and cover the pot with a lid sitting upside down.

5. Place ice in the pot's upside-down lid.

6. Let the pot simmer on medium heat for about twenty minutes. Replace the ice in the lid as it melts.

7. The vapor in the pot will condense on the underside of the lid and drip into the bowl. Once the bowl is filled with hydrosol, set it aside and let it cool.

8. Pour into a glass container for storage.

PRETTY ROSE HYDROSOL

Quantity can vary

1½ cups dried rose petals or buds
or 4 cups fresh, pesticide-free rose petals

Ice

Large stock pot with lid

Metal bowl or heat-safe glass bowl

Spray bottle or spritz bottle

Place rose petals/buds in the pot. If you are using fresh flowers, make sure the petals and buds are pushed down into the water. Add enough water to completely cover the petals, and bring the pot to a simmer.

In the pot, place a strainer or other item that will support a bowl. The purpose is to keep the bowl from touching the bottom of the pot. Some people use a clean brick for this, however I prefer a metal strainer. Place the bowl on the strainer—or whatever support you use—and cover the pot with a lid, positioned upside down. Place ice into the upside-down lid.

Simmer for about 30 minutes, replacing the ice as it melts. The vapor in the pot will condense on the underside of the lid and drip into the bowl. Once the bowl is filled with the rose hydrosol, set it aside and let it cool completely. Pour into container for storage until you use. I prefer a glass or BPA-free container with a lid. If using alone as a toner, pour the rose hydrosol into a spray bottle or any bottle that can be used by easily applying to a cotton ball.

When to Discard: about 6 months

OIL INFUSIONS

Although infusions can be created with water or oil, only oil infusions will be discussed in this chapter because oil-type ingredients are preferred in this book's recipes. An infused oil is a carrier oil that has been permeated or "infused" with plant material such as herbs or flowers. When plant material is seeped in oil for a certain amount of time, it allows the oil to absorb the properties of the plant.

Herbs contain medicinal properties that can be very beneficial for the skin when infused in oils. Infusions allow for a lot of creativity for combining various ingredients. Different herbs and flowers offer different benefits and contribute different scents to your recipes. The infused oil is then used alone or combined with other ingredients to make the perfect combination of plant extracts and nourishing oils.

There are two ways to make an oil infusion: the quick heat method or a slower solar method.

Quick Heat Method:

1. In a slow-cooker or stovetop pot, place herbs and a carrier oil of your choice.

2. Completely cover herbs with oil, leaving an inch or two at the top.

3. Gently heat the herbs on *very* low heat (approximately 120°F) for thirty minutes to four hours, until the oil takes on the color and scent desired.

4. Some experts recommend heating the oil overnight in a slow-cooker on the lowest setting.

5. Turn off heat and allow to completely cool.

6. Strain out the herbs using a cheesecloth.

7. Bottle the infusion in dry, sterilized glass bottles with a lid.

1. Pack herbs in a clean, dry canning jar, leaving at least an inch of space at the top.

2. Fill the jar with a carrier oil of your choice; cover the herbs with at least one inch of oil.

3. Use a canning weight to keep herbs below oil.

4. Cap the jar tightly.

5. Place jar in a sunny, warm windowsill. Gently shake once a day.

6. After two to four weeks, strain the herbs out of the oil using cheesecloth or a mesh strainer.

7. Bottle the infusion in dry, sterilized glass bottles with a lid.

GREEN TEA & COFFEE INFUSED OIL

Makes 4 ounces

> 1 tablespoon loose leaf green tea
>
> 1 tablespoon unused coffee grounds
>
> ¼ cup grapeseed oil
>
> 1 tablespoon almond extract (oil-based)

Place grapeseed oil, green tea and coffee grounds in a pot on your stove. Gently warm on very low heat, stirring frequently for about one hour, until the oil takes on the color and scent desired. Turn off heat and allow the infusion to completely cool.

Strain using a cheesecloth and then stir in almond extract. Bottle in sterilized glass bottles.

When to Discard: about 6–8 months depending on shelf life of carrier oil

ALCOHOL TINCTURES

Tinctures are concentrated herbal extracts that often have grain alcohol as the solvent. Some herbalists will use glycerin or vinegar for certain tinctures as well. For the tinctures in this book, we are using a full-strength alcohol without the addition of water or another liquid. Often tinctures are diluted with other liquids, such as water, to obtain the correct strength. However, the tinctures in this book are a higher concentration and will be able to be used quicker than a diluted tincture.

Tinctures are extracts, but not all extracts are tinctures because not all of them contain alcohol. If vinegar, glycerin, or water—basically anything other than alcohol—are used in your preparation, it is an extract, not a tincture. Any type of alcohol can be used in tinctures. However, many herbalists prefer something more neutral, such as vodka, so the taste of the herb comes through.

In skin-care products, extracts and tinctures help balance the skin and add the therapeutic benefits of raw plant material to your recipes. Tinctures mix well with water-based ingredients such as aloe vera and witch hazel, making them great for toners or spot-treatment rollers.

How to Make a Tincture

The general rule is to use about 1 ounce of plant material per cup of alcohol.

1. Place plant material in a glass jar and fill remaining space with 80 proof (40%) alcohol.

2. Cover with a lid and set aside.

3. Gently shake the tincture every day for about one month. (You can leave it for up to three months.) Over this time, the alcohol will absorb the plant material.

4. After your infusion is complete, you should not be able to taste any alcohol.

5. Strain the plant material using cheesecloth, and transfer the tincture to a sealable, dark-colored container.

THE BENEFITS OF
WHITE WILLOW BARK

White willow bark is used quite often in skin care—and for good reason! There are both health and beauty benefits to using this wonderful bark. Willow bark comes from the low-growing, deciduous willow tree that has long, slender, green leaves. In the 1800s, chemist Felix Hoffmann discovered that the active ingredient salicin, from willow trees, could be used to relieve pain. He used this knowledge to create aspirin and then went on to found the Bayer company.

However, using willow bark for pain goes back even further in time. Around 460 to 377 BC, Hippocrates believed that chewing on willow bark in its pure form relieved pain and fevers. The ancient Egyptians also had several remedies containing willow bark concoctions.

Willow bark is used in natural skin-care formulas because of its natural content of salicylic acid. Salicylic acid can remove dead skin cells and help promote fresh, new cellular growth for a more youthful complexion. By using products containing willow bark, you can improve skin tone more naturally.

Willow bark also offers anti-inflammatory properties that can relieve skin swelling and sensitivity. This makes it ideal for conditions such as rosacea, cystic acne, and even aging skin. Willow bark can also minimize age spots and discoloration due to its mild exfoliating properties.

WHITE WILLOW BARK TINCTURE

Makes 8 ounces

Prep time: 2 to 4 weeks

> 1 cup vodka (40% alcohol or 80 proof)
>
> ½ cup dried and chopped willow bark*

Place chopped willow bark in a glass canning jar, then completely fill it with vodka. Use a canning weight to press down the bark to keep it from floating to the top. Close the lid on the jar and let sit in a warm, sunny place for 2 to 4 weeks, shaking it gently once a day. The longer the bark "marinates," the stronger it will be.

Use a cheesecloth to strain out the willow bark, leaving a potent tincture for use in the Acne-Clearing Vanilla Toner (page 48) and Blemish-Clearing Essential Oil Roller (page 172) recipes. Store in a dark-glass jar with a lid.

* You can purchase white willow bark online or at a local health food store.

When to Discard: about 2 years

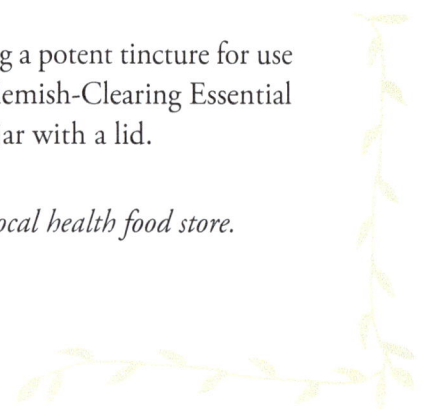

CALENDULA TINCTURE

Makes 8 ounces

Prep time: 4 to 5 weeks

Calendula has amazing benefits for the skin. It is most commonly used to reduce inflammation and irritation, which is helpful at calming acne and hydrating the skin.

> 1 cup vodka (40% alcohol or 80 proof)

> ½ cup dried calendula flowers

Place calendula flowers in a glass canning jar, then completely fill it with vodka. Use a canning weight to press down the flowers to keep them from floating to the top. Close the lid on the jar and let it sit in a warm, sunny place for 4 to 5 weeks, shaking it gently once a day. The longer the calendula "marinates," the stronger it will be.

Use a cheesecloth to strain out the calendula, leaving a potent tincture for use in the Blemish-Clearing Essential Oil Roller (page 172). Store in a dark-glass jar with a lid.

When to Discard: about 2 years

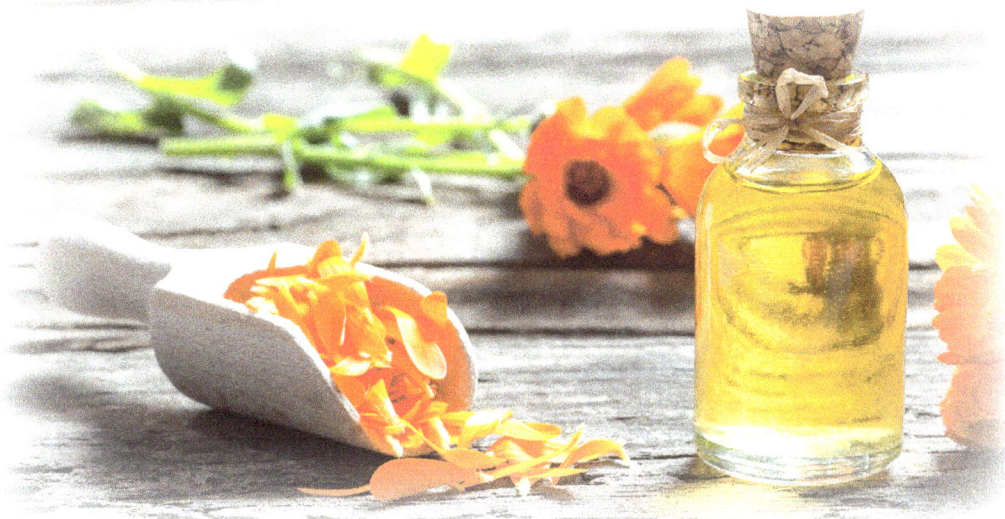

FENNEL TINCTURE

Makes 8 ounces

Prep time: 2 to 3 weeks

1 cup vodka (40% alcohol or 80 proof)

¼ cup dried fennel seeds

Place fennel in a glass canning jar, then completely fill it with vodka. Use a canning weight to press down the seeds to keep them from floating to the top. Close the lid on the jar and let it sit in a warm, sunny place for 2 to 3 weeks, shaking it gently once a day. The longer the fennel "marinates," the stronger it will be.

Use a cheesecloth to strain out the herbs, leaving a potent tincture for use in facial toners, such as the Soothing Fennel Balance Toner on page 48. Store in a dark-glass jar with a lid.

When to Discard: about 2 years

MINTY BREATH FRESHENER

Makes 4 ounces

This handy breath freshener is a great alternative to standard breath mints, which can contain a lot of added sugars and harmful ingredients. Not only that, the ingredients in this spray are actually GOOD for you!

Prep time: 3 to 4 weeks

1 tablespoon dried mint leaves

1 teaspoon dried minced ginger root

1 tablespoon dried fennel

1 teaspoon dried cinnamon powder

3-5 whole cloves

½ cup high-quality vodka or rum
(40% alcohol or 80 proof)*

1 teaspoon peppermint or cinnamon food-grade
flavor or extract (optional)

Place herbs and spices in a glass canning jar, then completely fill it with vodka. Use a canning weight to keep everything from floating to the top. Close the lid on the jar and let it sit in a cool, dark area for 3 to 4 weeks, shaking it gently once a day. The longer the mixture "marinates," the stronger it will be.

Use a cheesecloth to strain out the herbs. Add peppermint or cinnamon (flavor or extract) if desired. Place in a small spritz bottle or small glass bottle with a dropper. Use as needed.

* If you infuse the mixture long enough, the alcohol will be diminished and only the herb flavor should remain. Use a high-quality alcohol since you will be spraying this in your mouth.

When to Discard: about a year

CHAPTER 17

Natural Solutions

FOR SKIN AILMENTS

The four main skin conditions that my clients have questions about are acne, large pores, eczema, and rosacea. Since these are the most common ailments, I am focusing on them the most but that is not to say there are not several other concerns that clients have. Here are a number of other issues that frequently come up, along with some natural suggestions for clearing them up.

Common Skin Ailments		
Type	**Symptoms**	**Natural Remedy**
Melasma	Much like hyperpigmentation, melasma causes dark patches on the forehead, bridge of the nose, chin and/or upper lip area, but these patches can appear anywhere. It's often called "the mask of pregnancy" because hormones can cause dark facial patches that can look mask-like. Melasma can be caused by hormones and excessive sun exposure. It is more apparent on those with darker skin tones.	Avoid excess sun exposure, increase vitamins C and E. Products such as apple cider vinegar, turmeric, lactic acid, lemon and aloe can be helpful topically. **Suggested Recipes:** Honey-Coconut Facial Scrub (p. 43), Simple Brightening Lemon Toner (p. 47), Vitamin C Boost Serum (p. 85), Brightening Turmeric Glow Mask (p. 68), Skin Repair & Balance Smoothie (p. 193)

Common Skin Ailments		
Type	**Symptoms**	**Natural Remedy**
Vitiligo	The dictionary states that vitiligo is a condition in which pigment is lost from areas of the skin, causing whitish patches. There's often no clear cause. Vitiligo occurs when pigment-producing cells actually stop functioning, and there is no known cure.	Topical turmeric masks can help with discoloration. Eating foods rich in beta-carotene, vitamin B12, zinc, and folic acid also help. Ginkgo biloba has also been found to be effective. It is important to manage your stress as it may contribute to the problem. Lemon and citrus fruits are *not* recommended. **Suggested Recipe:** Brightening Turmeric Glow Mask (p. 68)
Hyperpigmentation	This darkening of the skin in certain areas can be caused by excess sun, aging, and/or a post-inflammatory response to an injury (such as acne). Hyperpigmentation is an excess of melanin, the brown pigment that produces normal skin color, when it forms deposits on the skin.	Natural skin brightening remedies can be helpful, including apple cider vinegar, lemon, aloe vera, and turmeric. **Suggested Recipes:** Light Aloe Facial Moisturizer (p. 99), Simple Brightening Lemon Toner (p. 47), Vitamin C Boost Serum (p. 85), Brightening Turmeric Glow Mask (p. 68)

Common Skin Ailments		
Type	**Symptoms**	**Natural Remedy**
Cellulite	This esthetic condition is caused by an imbalance of connective tissue, and it appears on certain areas of the body, especially the thighs. Cellulite causes a dimpling of the skin.	Regular exercise and improving lymph drainage is very helpful. There are several topical things to try, which can smooth out the skin. Gentle massage with a body scrub can minimize the appearance of cellulite. Detox baths and diet are also effective. **Suggested Recipes:** Cinnamon-Coffee Body Scrub (p. 58), Sweet Red Body Scrub (p. 63), Oil-Balancing Sea-Salt Scrub (p. 60), Refreshing Peppermint Bath Salts (p. 112), Lymph-Drainage Massage (p. 36)
Acne	Inflamed or infected oil glands, also known as pimples. When referred to as acne, it is more commonly understood as persistent infected areas covering a large area that can be painful and uncomfortable. Minor breakouts are common for most people, but acne is more extreme. Further discussion in the following section.	See the section that starts on page 166 for more information on acne. **Suggested Recipes:** Gentle Acne Facial Cleanser (p. 44), Activated Charcoal Skin-Clearing Mask (p. 73), Acne-Clearing Vanilla Toner (p. 48), Blemish-Clearing Essential Oil Roller (p. 172), Skin Repair & Balance Smoothie (p. 193)

Common Skin Ailments		
Large Pores	Large pores are often visible to the naked eye. It is common to have larger pores if you have oily skin and/or are prone to acne or breakouts. As we age, pores become larger and more prominent as well. Additionally, clogged pores can look larger than clean pores.	See the section that starts on page 173 for more information on large pores. **Suggested Recipes:** Honey-Coconut Facial Scrub (p. 43), Young & Refreshed Facial Steam (p. 51), Activated Charcoal Skin-Clearing Mask (p. 73), Deep-Cleansing Clay Mask (p. 70)
Eczema	Eczema commonly shows up as itchy red patches. However, some breakouts can blister, weep, or peel. Alternately, eczema can be dry and scaly. The most common type of eczema is atopic dermatitis.	See the section that starts on page 174 for more information on eczema. **Suggested Recipes:** Nice & Gentle Skin Oil (p. 101), Kid-Friendly Moisturizing Mask (p. 71)
Rosacea	Symptoms of rosacea often include a flushed, red face with sensitive, dry skin that may burn or sting. Redness can be on the nose, cheeks, chin, and forehead. Small bumps may be present, often with swelling and pimples. Some people experience fine red lines and/or acne-like breakouts.	See the section that starts on page 180 for more information on rosacea. **Suggested Recipes:** Hydrating Olive Oil Cleanser (p. 41), Kid-Friendly Moisturizing Mask (p. 71)

WAYS TO IMPROVE ACNE

Acne is the most frustrating skin issue clients have. What is surprising is that many of my clients who suffer from persistent acne are *not* teenagers. Teenagers do get acne, however, with proper care and a healthier diet, they are often able to get their skin to improve. Young adults suffering from acne tend to have persistent acne without much relief. This is often due to hormones that are out of balance or chronic stress.

First, it is important to remember that if you suffer from acne it is probably not your fault. Acne occurs when the skin's oil glands produce too much oil. As a result, skin follicles get clogged and the over-oily skin allows naturally occurring bacteria to go haywire. Sometimes the skin can feel or appear very dry even with an overproduction of oil, because the skin is imbalanced. The result is whiteheads, blackheads, and inflammation. Oil "overload" can clog hair follicles where bacteria grows and cause acne to form. Additionally, acne (and minor breakouts) in women can come and go in response to the "monthly visitor."

For moderate to severe acne, it may be best to discuss different options with your physician or a trusted dermatologist. Sometimes a low-dose birth control pill or an acne-type medication is prescribed to help regulate hormone levels and reduce acne symptoms. Sometimes these remedies can be helpful. However, I personally choose to focus on natural remedies and leave prescriptions as a last resort.

Research has shown that despite the many myths about what causes acne—diet, poor hygiene, and the body's overall hormone levels—these are not always the culprits. With so much mystery surrounding the cause, it is reasonable to suspect genetics. It seems logical that parents could pass down skin that over-produces oil, just like they can pass down genes for red hair and blue eyes. Recent studies have found that the greater the number of family members with acne, the more likely a teen will also develop acne, especially if the teen's mother had a history of acne.

One thing to keep in mind is that your skin is constantly regenerating itself. It takes about a month to see the full results of repaired skin once your skin begins to heal itself.

Have a Facial Cleansing Routine

One reason I push skin-care routines is that they help to balance the skin and therefore minimize acne. See more about facial routines in Chapter 4. Washing with a *mild* cleanser (not soap) every morning and every evening before bed will help. Do not skip a face-wash before bedtime. Ever. Washing your face before turning in for the night is most important as your skin cells are rejuvenating themselves as you sleep. Take this opportunity to allow your skin to repair itself. Use a mild toner, (such as witch hazel or the Fennel Toner on page 48), after cleansing.

Use a light, moisturizing facial cream after each cleansing routine in both the evening and in the morning to help balance the skin's oils. Sometimes it is helpful to put on a nourishing oil serum with acne-fighting properties before bedtime.

Eat an Anti-Acne Diet

Drink plenty of water daily, and avoid junk food, especially foods high in sugar. Fill your diet with fruits, vegetables, and protein. Think of repairing your skin like a stoplight: *Stop* and begin adding in healthy vegetables and fruits in red, yellow/orange, and green colors to begin repair as soon as possible. Avoid unnatural additives and processed foods. If you love dairy, look for organic foods without hormones (rBST). Try shredding your own organic cheese (hard cheeses are best) and avoid soft, processed cheese. Limit your intake of fat, caffeine, and sugar.

Red - watermelon, tomatoes, beets and red peppers

Yellow/Orange - carrots, cantaloupe, oranges and sweet potatoes

Green - leafy greens, avocado, green beans, cucumbers and green tea

To help repair your skin, eat fruits and vegetables that are red, yellow/orange, and green.

Keep Your Face Clean

Oils and bacteria can be spread or increase with the touch of your fingertips, so avoid touching your face or holding your head up with your hand. Also, try not to constantly have your phone smashed to your face, which could cause breakouts in that area.

Hair can add to unnecessary oils on your face as well, so it helps to keep your hair off your face, especially at night. Pin it back or pull it into a ponytail while sleeping. Also, beware of too much hair product. Excess hair sprays and other hair products can cause an acne flareup if your hair is often touching your face.

It sounds crazy, but it is also important to wash your pillowcase often. Oil and dirt from your skin can build up on the pillowcase and cause breakouts. Likewise, don't forget to clean your makeup brushes regularly.

CLEAN YOUR MAKEUP BRUSHES

Anyone who loves makeup gets super excited about a fresh new set of makeup brushes. New brushes feel so great when putting on make-up. However, many of us busy ladies forget to clean them. It may not seem like a big deal to keep brushes clean, but many breakouts can be blamed on these bacteria-infested bristles.

Frequently used makeup brushes retain old makeup, and they also hold on to oils and bacteria from your skin, which can cause clogged pores and irritation. A simple solution is to keep your brushes clean. Any time you begin to see residue on the tips of your bristles is a good time to give them a good wash. Cleaning your brushes helps keep your skin clear and also will increase the life of your brush. This is especially important if you purchase higher quality brushes.

How to Clean Your Brushes

There are many cleaning solutions made specifically for makeup brush-es. However, I like to use a simple recipe or cleanser I already own. Al-though any gentle, natural face wash will work, I use one of the Green Eyed Grace Gentle cleansers to wash them. You can also use a gentle castile soap on dirty brushes. To do this, place castile soap into a little glass jar and submerge your brushes (brush-side down) until they are well covered by soap. Massage the soap into the bristles, and rinse thoroughly with warm water.

Be sure to press out any excess water from the bristles. I like to let mine air-dry on a clean hand towel for several hours. Do *not* stand your brushes straight up right after cleaning. Doing so will cause excess water to settle at the base of the brush, which could create unwanted bacteria. I usually shake out my brush to remove as much water from the bristles as possible before I lay them on the towel.

Be sure to keep brushes in a space where they will stay clean—like a pretty glass jar or their own pouch. Avoid throwing brushes into a drawer or makeup bag where they can easily get dirty.

Stay Out of the Sun

The sun causes the most damage to your skin by accelerating aging. Additionally, the sun can be drying and cause an acne flareup. Avoid excess sunlight, and if you do plan to spend a day at the beach or pool, stay in the shade, wear a hat, and be sure to protect yourself with sunscreen.

What You Should Know about Extractions

Unfortunately, we do not talk enough about doing extractions, also known as "popping zits." As teens we are told to leave our face alone, but no one does. Without knowing how to properly extract your own blemishes, scarring can occur.

Types of Zits	
Whiteheads	· Non-inflammatory · Not very painful · White-colored pore
Blackheads	· Non-inflammatory · Open comedones · Small black or dark-colored pore · Trapped dirt
Papules/Pustules	· Inflamed bump under skin · Swollen · Often filled with pus
Nodules/Cysts	· Deeper inflamed bump under skin · Painful · Cannot always extract

If you are suffering from nodular or cystic acne, it is best to see a trusted esthetician or dermatologist. Doing extraction may cause more trouble for your skin. However, it is still important to have a good skin-care routine and eat healthy. Both will be beneficial.

A helpful tip about extractions is to wait until you see the white! Once a blemish comes "to a head" it is okay to "pop" it, but very gently. Treat your skin like you would a baby—nice and gentle. Do not tear your skin under any circumstance—this can cause scarring. Some blemishes will disappear on their own, but if you want to try to extract the bacteria, do so very carefully.

A WORD ON MILIA

Milia is a medical term used by dermatologists to describe the tiny white bumps that periodically occur on the face. They can either be found in a little cluster (milia), or you may only have one little loner (a millium). These are not white-heads but a hard, tiny keratin cyst that is sealed up as tight as a submarine door.

Trying to get milia out can damage the skin because they are so stubborn. Having an esthetician or a dermatologist professionally remove them is the safest route. Milia form when the skin has trouble naturally exfoliating. Dead skin cells are composed primarily of keratin, a protein also found in hair and nails. Milia result from dead skin-cell buildup, which causes a tiny bump to form.

That being said, regular, gentle exfoliation can help keep these stubborn bumps at bay. The Coconut-Lemon Sugar Scrub (page 59) is an excellent product that helps soften the skin and prevent these bumps. The honey helps to nourish the skin, while the sugar gently sloughs away dead skin cells. Another important factor in avoiding these little white bumps is to avoid overexposure to the sun. Hardened, sun-damaged skin is more susceptible to developing milia.

The most important step in doing extractions is to start with a clean face. Use a toner after the extraction to clean the affected area. Ever wonder why when you pop a zit, the next day you have another zit right next to it? This is usually because the bacteria that came out of the first blemish remained on the skin, causing a new blemish. Therefore, it is important to make sure the entire area is clean before *and* after you have done the extraction.

Another important tip is to lift blemishes from the side, not the top. It is easy to assume if you take the tip off the top, you can squeeze out the pus and bacteria. However, this tears the skin, which often will not heal properly. If you make a tiny hole from the side with a sterile lancet (like those used to prick your finger in a doctor's office), you can gently extract bacteria and allow the skin to lie back down, healing properly. It is important to not overdo it. If you make a tiny hole and nothing comes out, you may be dealing with a nodule or a cyst and it is best to leave it alone.

ACNE BLEMISH

hair follicle

inflammation

Gently lift from the side, not the top

bacteria

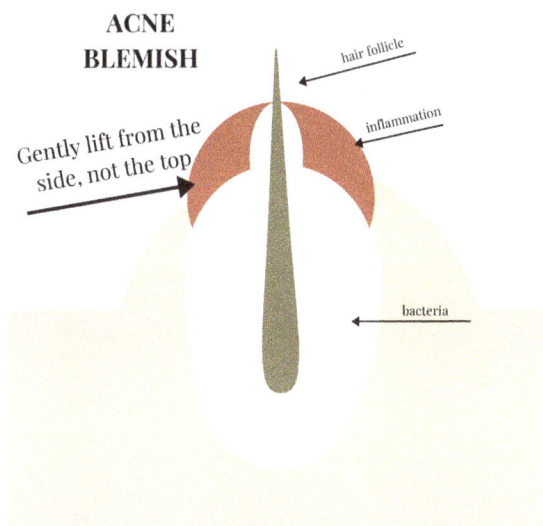

Anatomy of a pimple

Raw honey has natural antiseptic properties that can be very effective at treating breakouts. Honey can bring a blemish to a "head." Dab a little raw honey on pimples and let it sit overnight. This only works well for one or two blemishes as it can be sticky. You do not want to be glued to your pillowcase in the morning, so use sparingly. To make your own honey mask, try the Honey-Oat Hydrating Mask recipe on page 67.

BENEFITS OF TEA TREE (MELALEUCA)

Tea tree oil is widely used in skin care, and for good reason. This healing oil is effective in treating various skin troubles, including acne, dandruff, and skin rashes. It has natural antiseptic and anti-inflammatory benefits, making it a fundamental beauty necessity.

Tea tree oil, also known as melaleuca oil, is made from steam distillation of leaves from the Melaleuca alternifolia plant. This tree or shrub is part of the myrtle family, which is native to Australia. It has a crisp, camphorous odor and has been used throughout Australia for centuries. Numerous medical studies have shown that tea tree oil eliminates many strains of bacteria, viruses, and fungi. It is also well known for its powerful antiseptic properties and ability to treat wounds.

Tea tree oil is helpful with treating psoriasis, sores, boils, and sunburns. However, it is most commonly used on acne and breakouts because it is highly effective. Pimples can easily become infected or inflamed, but applying tea tree oil can help eliminate bacteria and heal the skin.

BLEMISH-CLEARING ESSENTIAL OIL ROLLER

Makes 10 milliters

I started making "zit zappers" for a few clients who were struggling with break-outs between facials. They are a quick and easy way to treat an area headed for a breakout or where one has already happened. Often we get one annoying zit after having too much pizza or being in the hot sun too long during summer vacation. With a handy blemish roller, you can quickly clear up these little breakouts. Keep one in your purse or makeup bag to use any time you need it.

> 1 teaspoon vodka
>
> 1 teaspoon witch hazel
>
> ⅛ dropper of calendula tincture*
>
> ⅛ dropper of infused white willow bark tincture** (optional)
>
> 4 drops tea tree essential oil
>
> 3 drops lemon essential oil
>
> 2 drops frankincense essential oil

Combine all ingredients in a measuring cup or small container and transfer to a 10 ml roller using a small funnel. If you do not like to measure, pour vodka into a glass essential oil roller until it is about half full. (I like to use the little metal essential oil funnels for less mess.) Pour witch hazel into the essential oil roller and fill it *almost* to the top. Add the calendula tincture and essential oils. Press on the cap, and give it a gentle shake.

Roll on itchy areas that could potentially be a breakout or where already troubled skin needs treatment. You can make your own tinctures as referenced below or you can purchase pre-made tinctures online from Amazon.com or natural health food stores.

* To make your own Calendula Tincture, see page 159.

** To make your own White Willow Bark Tincture, see page 158.

When to Discard: about 8 months

WAYS TO MINIMIZE LARGE PORES

I have clients who complain about their 'extremely' large pores on a weekly basis. What is interesting is that rarely do they have abnormally large pores. As we get older, our pores naturally become larger. Additionally, if you have oily skin, you will most likely have larger pores. This is nothing to be embarrassed about. Many clients who come in with tiny pores usually have very dry, tight skin. Having larger pores and oily skin is more flattering, hands down. So first things first: embrace larger pores because it means your skin is working properly.

That being said, there are a few ways to help minimize large pores. The first is having a daily skin-care regimen that includes consistent cleansing, toning, and moisturizing. (I am sure you are no longer surprised by this suggestion!) More importantly, try to exfoliate about three times per week. Exfoliating really helps clean out pores and stimulates the skin to have an overall better tenacity.

Avoid a cleanser that is too harsh, and avoid a moisturizer that is too heavy. Consistently squeezing pores can make them look larger. Instead, try using a rotating brush to clean your pores. Another thing that is helpful is to never sleep in your makeup or skip your cleansing routine. This can create an imbalance and cause oil glands to overproduce oil, creating larger pores.

Additionally, if you wear makeup, try using a primer under your makeup to minimize the appearance of pores and help makeup stay in place. Apply foundation in light layers with a sponge and change out the sponge often—like every other day. Avoid too much foundation as it will bring attention to the pores. Other helpful tips include applying foundation in downward strokes and avoiding any shimmer in a foundation or powder. Finish your makeup by using a pressed powder, and use a cheek stain or a blush that does not contain shimmer. Apply blotting papers throughout the day to remove excess oil.

WAYS TO IMPROVE ECZEMA

This is where it all began for me. Fighting eczema is the whole reason I became so passionate about healthier skin care and clean ingredients. Eczema is a very common skin ailment that can be very difficult to correct. If you add in chemical-type products to that equation, clearing up the skin becomes even more difficult.

What Is Eczema?

Eczema can show up in many different ways on the skin—most commonly as itchy red patches. However, some breakouts can blister, weep or be flaky, dry, and/or scaly. The most common type of eczema is atopic dermatitis, which generally refers to the type that can be linked to heredity. Often this type of eczema can exist in combination with other allergic conditions, such as asthma and hay fever.

Eczema can be one of the most frustrating skin issues for estheticians because there can be so many reasons (internally and externally) for a flare-up. Consequently, it can take a while to get the outbreak under control and begin to reverse the irritation. Many people who suffer from eczema become very frustrated or feel like living with eczema is just a way of life. This does not have to be the case. There is always a reason for the problem and always a solution that will work. Patience and having the correct remedy is the key. Keep in mind that symptoms and solutions can be different for everyone.

Improve Your Diet

Skin problems are not always linked to something we put on our skin. Often there is a deeper problem. What we put into our bodies is reflected in our skin. More than likely, this is the case with eczema. A breakout can be triggered by foods that your body may be rejecting. You may have an allergy to a certain food or perhaps an overload of processed foods, alcohol, or medications.

Start eating a diet full of fruits and vegetables, which are high in antioxidants. The more color the better. Avoid processed foods, excessive sugar, and "fake" sugar. Soda pop and energy drinks can be full of harmful ingredients, so read your labels. My rule of thumb is that if you do not recognize a word as a real food ingredient (such as maltodextrin, dextrose, high-fructose corn syrup, trisodium phosphate) do not buy it.

> *"What we put into our bodies is reflected in our skin."*

—Bethel Jiricek

Reduce Stress

Eczema is a nerve-related disorder. Sometimes it is your body's way of letting you know there is a problem. If you suffer from anxiety, you may be more prone to an eczema breakout. If you believe this may be the reason for the problem, try to eliminate stress and take care of yourself by getting a massage, venting to a loved one, praying, meditating or doing yoga.

Balance Your Hormones

Believe it or not, hormones can also play a role in eczema. Sometimes women will see a difference in their eczema around the time of menstruation. If you believe hormones are an issue, try to eliminate dairy products with rBST and buy organic. This may help. Organic milk and organic Greek yogurt with no added hormones are best if you love your dairy products. Balancing herbs such as raspberry tea, rhodiola, ashwaganda, holy basil, and cinnamon can also be helpful.

Be Choosy about Skin-Care Products

Your personal-care products can also cause problems when it comes to your skin. Chemicals in products will eventually take a toll on your skin. Avoid products that have a lot of ingredients that are hard to understand. Stick to natural, soft soaps and cleansers, and after you bathe, put a pure oil (such as an oil listed on page 178) on your skin instead of a lotion.

Be Savvy about Household Products

One eczema factor that gets overlooked is your laundry detergent. Washing your clothes in a detergent riddled with chemicals and/or bleach can be very irritating to the skin. Try using a "free and clear" detergent, or make your own. Even some of the "free and clear" detergents can be irritating. Also, wearing new clothes, scarves, or coats without washing them first can cause an outbreak of eczema. Anything that touches your skin can also irritate your skin.

Keep Pets Out of Your Bed

We love our pets, but if you have a dander allergy, playing with an animal can cause an eczema flare-up. You may try to lessen the amount of time your skin comes in contact with your pet's fur. Also, if pets sleep on your bed or sofa, it could cause irritation to your skin because that is where you spend much of your time. Try protecting the couch or bed with a sheet, or no longer let pets hang out there. Easier said than done, I know!

Monitor Your Allergies

Those prone to seasonal allergies or who have a family history of allergies are more likely to suffer from eczema. Sometimes being aware of things you need to avoid can help improve breakouts. You may find that once you have changed your diet and removed chemical-type products from your home, you will experience fewer allergy symptoms.

Beat the Heat

One of the worst eczema breakouts my son had as an infant was when he was in his car seat for a long ride. The weather was very hot, and even with air conditioning, the car was not staying cool enough. If you are unable to avoid the heat, try wearing breathable cotton fabrics whenever possible.

How to Start Making Changes

Start with personal-care products and detergents then move to food and so on. It can be easy to get overwhelmed, so start slow. One thing to consider if you are an adult and suffering from an eczema outbreak but have not had an outbreak in a very long time, is that it could be your body's way of raising a red flag. There may be more going on inside than you know, such as an illness that needs attention. If you feel this may be the case, you will want to get a blood test and see a well-respected physician.

If you have an infant or child suffering from eczema, keep in mind that many babies outgrow eczema and other unexplained breakouts like cradle cap. Eczema in infants and children can be uncomfortable for them and cause bad sleep habits. Getting professional help is important if natural remedies do not help.

SMOOTH-CAP SCALP TREATMENT FOR YOUNG ONES

Makes enough for one use

I used this handy recipe on my son when he was fighting cradle cap. I do not recommend using this on small infants because it can be a little bit abrasive if not massaged gently. I suggest this recipe for infants and children ages six months and older.

3 tablespoons pure, unrefined, raw coconut oil

1 teaspoon baking soda

Water

Combine ingredients. Add a few drops of water and gently massage into scalp using circular motions. Rinse thoroughly. Repeat if necessary.

When to Discard: Use immediately; do not store.

Finding Replacement Products

Many of us who suffer from eczema have found that everyday products (lotions, cleansers, laundry detergent) are causing skin irritation, yet sometimes changing products does not give us the results we hope for. Additionally, trying to find replacement products with fewer harmful chemicals is usually pretty difficult. Petroleum-based products, such as Vaseline, are a popular lotion replacement because they are easy on the skin, have minimal ingredients, and are somewhat effective at temporarily clearing up eczema. However, petroleum-based products do not allow your skin to breathe properly, and they are suspected to be carcinogenic. So, instead of turning to a product that may be harmful to your health, a DIY recipe or pure body oils might be a better solution.

NATURAL BODY OILS TO USE INSTEAD OF LOTION

- Almond oil
- Apricot kernel oil
- Avocado oil
- Calendula oil
- Carrot seed oil
- Castor oil

- Chamomile oil
- Coconut oil
- Evening primrose oil
- Grapeseed oil
- Jojoba oil
- Olive oil

- Pomegranate seed oil
- Rosehip seed oil
- Safflower oil
- Sea buckthorn oil
- Sesame oil
- Sunflower oil

Other Topical Treatments

Aloe vera: Straight from the plant is best. Aloe is known to assist healing of skin and wounds. It is also favored by many as an effective sunburn remedy.

Cocoa butter: Naturally contains beneficial nutrients that can benefit your skin. It is important to buy cocoa butter in its most pure form. Apply right after bathing for best results. A note of caution: some may find cocoa butter slightly irritating because of its gritty texture.

Coconut oil: Raw, unrefined coconut oil can be effective due to its anti-inflammatory properties. Applying coconut oil to your skin can improve hydration and is a wonderful replacement for mineral oil. Its nourishing properties have been known to heal and treat eczema. However, in some cases, coconut oil can be irritating for those who suffer from eczema. In that case, having coconut oil in your regular diet is a great alternative. Try using it in your smoothies and heal from the inside out.

Carrots: Carrots can be puréed to a juice and mixed in with aloe vera to calm and nourish the skin. Additionally, try using carrot seed oil. Carrots have soothing properties, beneficial nutrients for the skin, and they can help with itchiness.

Eczema can be a very frustrating skin problem. My advice is to keep looking for solutions. Do not give up! Gentle products and a clean environment, free of toxins, is a great place to start. Keeping a journal to track flare-up patterns can help pinpoint food allergies and triggers that are causing irritation.

CARROT SEED OIL

When you hear someone talking about carrot seed oil, they could be referring to one of two things: carrot seed carrier oil or carrot seed essential oil. The references to carrot seed oil in this book are referring to carrot seed carrier oil, which is a wonderfully rich oil that works well in skin care. Here are the differences:

Carrot Seed Carrier Oil: Produced through the cold-pressing of carrot seeds to create a vegetable-type oil. Carrot seed carrier oil is often used in skin care, and there are many great reasons to include this beautifully rich oil in your products. To say it is antioxidant rich is putting it lightly.

Carrot Seed Essential Oil: Produced through steam distillation of carrot seeds to create a concentrated oil.

Benefits:

- Carrot seed oil in general is full of nutrients such as beta-carotene and vitamins A and E.

- Both types of carrot seed oil are rich in carotenoids. Carotenoids protect the skin from sun damage and reverse damage caused by UV rays such as dark spots and sagging skin. In fact, studies have shown that carrot seed carrier oil can act as a natural SPF, although the percentage of SPF is unclear. With its deep, rich golden color it also naturally gives the skin a beautiful glow.

- Carrot seed oil can be a great under-eye oil for reducing puffiness and dark circles. It helps to reduce water retention and minimize dark spots.

- It helps improve skin tone, making carrot seed oil a great anti-aging ingredient for skin-care products.

WAYS TO HELP ROSACEA

Rosacea is a common skin disease that affects men and women over the age of thirty. Rosacea is most common on the face, affecting the T-zone area and the cheeks. Unfortunately, professionals are still unable to pinpoint a definite cause, and doctors do not believe there is a cure. However, there are many ways to control flare-ups and live a virtually rosacea-free life.

Symptoms of rosacea often include a flushed, red face with sensitive, dry skin that may burn or sting. Redness can be on the nose, cheeks, chin, and forehead. Small bumps may be present, often with swelling and pimples. Some people experience fine, red lines and/or acne-like breakouts. In more extreme cases rhinophyma can happen, which is an enlarged, sometimes bulbous, red nose. The skin gets coarser and thicker, with a bumpy texture. Dry, red, sore, or irritated eyes or conjunctivitis can also be present.

Rosacea tends to affect those who have fair skin or blush easily. Heredity can also play a role. Rosacea is not caused by alcohol abuse, as originally believed, although alcohol *can* trigger a flare-up of symptoms.

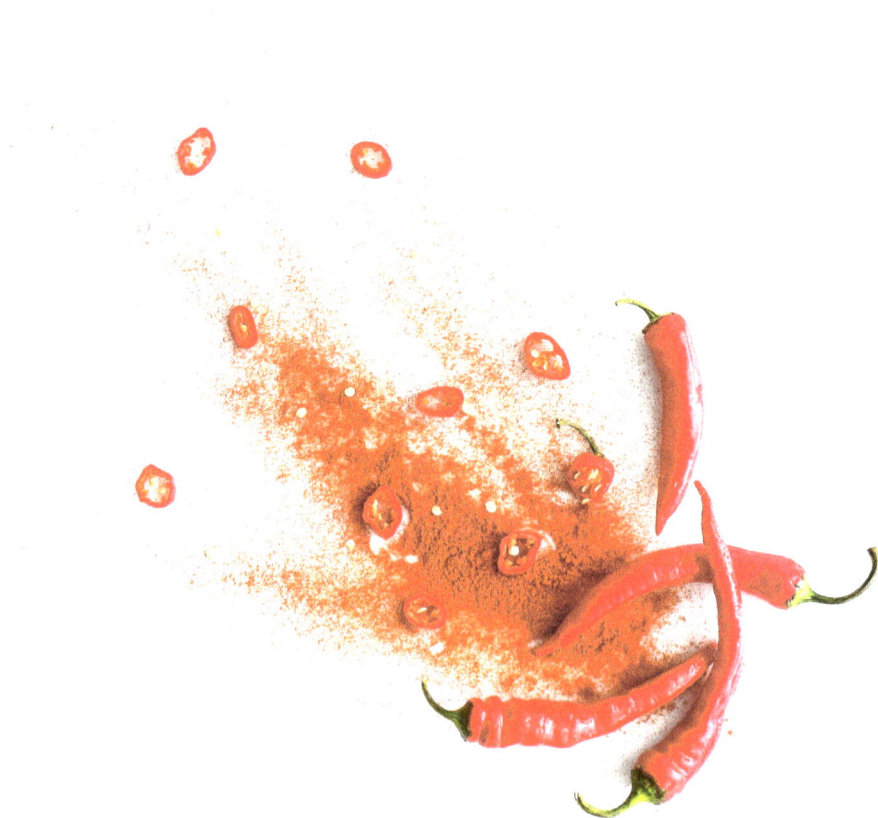

Triggers of Rosacea	Remedy
Sun	Protect your skin by staying out of the sun between peak hours (10 a.m. to 4 p.m.). When you are outdoors, protect your face by wearing a wide-brimmed hat, and apply a natural sunscreen that is free of chemicals.
Excessive wind exposure	Wear protective gear over your face, such as a cotton wind/face mask designed for snowboarders or other outdoor sports. Wear a good moisturizer before and after wind exposure.
Hot weather or extreme temperatures	Avoid overheating, especially on hot, summer days. Drink plenty of water and stay cool indoors or in the shade as much as possible.
Stress	Talk to a loved one about your stress, get regular facials and massages, try out yoga. Participate in activities you love that help relieve stress.
Spicy foods and alcohol	These particular triggers can be frustrating because food and an occasional glass of wine often bring joy to a person's life and help reduce stress. However, if you know foods or alcohol trigger a redder face and make the rosacea worse, they are not worth it.
Hot baths, saunas, or hot tubs	Reduce your time in hot baths, saunas and hot tubs to only a few minutes. Avoid altogether if facial redness does not disappear after about 20 minutes.
Beauty products (including essential oils)	Try switching to jojoba oil as a substitute for your regular moisturizer. Use natural skin-care products for sensitive skin. Avoid any products containing harmful ingredients or chemicals that can irritate your skin.

Know your triggers and how to avoid them. Not all triggers are the same, and everyone is different. A licensed professional may suggest or prescribe treatments to reduce redness and any breakouts. Overall, it is important to be gentle with your skin. Avoid scrubbing or over exfoliating your skin.

If you experience irritated eyes, apply a warm, wet cloth several times a day. Try soaking the washcloth with a little bit of chamomile tea or eyebright tea. Eat healthy, alkaline meals and anti-inflammatory foods and herbs, such as ginger and turmeric, in your everyday diet. Reduce processed foods and sugar intake.

Rosacea can be tough to treat, but there are solutions. Sometimes keeping a diary of when flare-ups happen will help you pinpoint the causes and triggers.

CHAPTER 18

A Common-Sense Diet

FOR WHOLE-BODY WELLNESS

I have never been one to jump on the bandwagon, so when I kept hearing everyone talking about this or that detox, I ignored the conversation, especially when I saw friends or co-workers eager to suck down a "detox" powdered shake instead of real food. After doing a little research, I learned that some detox plans can indeed be too extreme, but it is not true for all of them. Initially, I did not understand that our bodies held on to toxins and parasites. I think my exact words were, "That's ridiculous."

I still resist some of the extreme beliefs about all the sludge that supposedly sits in our intestines. However, I now understand the importance of detoxing the body by eliminating everyday toxins that we consume in our diet, breath from unclean air, and drink in our treated water systems. Detoxification is especially important for people whose diet is full of chemically laden or processed foods or for those who are regularly exposed to environmental pollutants and toxic household cleaners.

I get that we may need to take extra-good care of our body and abstain from certain foods or drinks in order to get the body back to working at an optimum level. It makes sense

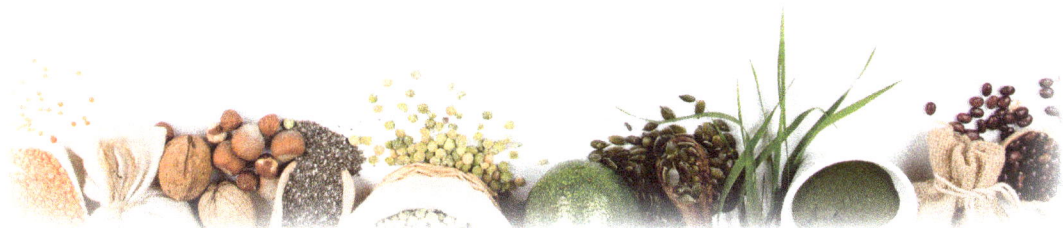

now! But what does *not* make sense to me is companies pushing products such as protein shakes, detox shakes, and synthetic vitamins that are full of preservatives and ingredients you cannot even pronounce and saying these products will help you detox. It also seems backward to deprive your body of nutrients in order to detox, especially if you are used to a certain type of diet. Depriving the body of foods it is used to seems like a terrible idea. So how do we know what detox program will work best? In this section I share some important lifestyle tips I have learned from working in a holistic environment and from the years of experience and research I have done on herbs, the body and health.

Take It Slow

Do not automatically stop eating solid foods and relying only on juice for nutrients. Extreme diets like this can make the body go into shock. Detoxing does not have to be extreme. This type of juice fast is not sustainable and can actually cause an adverse response when you finally cave in to your craving for food and then overeat or binge on high-sugar, high-carb foods because the cravings are so intense.

Know Your Body

If you know that your body craves carbohydrates and you are used to a high-carb diet, try not to cut out all carbs. Our bodies need healthy fats and nutrients from food in order to function. If you want to start cutting out carbs, do it gradually. It may be that you start with a detox plan that eliminates some types of carbs at first, with a long-term plan of having fewer carbs in your diet overall. This can also be the same for sugar, dairy, or other foods you are allergic to or that contribute to weight gain.

Make One Change at a Time

I find with herbs it is best to try one new thing at a time. When I feel like I have eaten too much junk food, I will drink a cup of dandelion tea, which really helps to improve digestive function and filter out toxins. Dandelion tea is kind of like my mini-detox. However, if I combine dandelion tea with any other detoxifying herb, I end up sending my stomach into turmoil and feel sick all night. It is better to take it slow.

WHY I LOVE DANDELION

One of the biggest marital arguments I have ever had was over dandelions! I want to protect them in our yard, and my husband wants to destroy them. It took many years of persuasion, but he has come to understand how much I love the dandelion—either that or has decided it is not worth the argument.

I don't just protect dandelions because they are a pretty flower, I guard them because they have so many health benefits. My favorite benefit, of course, is that they help the skin. Additionally, they are great when ingested for helping to cleanse the liver and kidneys. I try to enjoy a cup of dandelion root tea almost every day. It is a comfort to know all the benefits from just enjoying a cup of hot tea.

DANDELION'S BENEFITS

Organic dandelion is best because it is free of (or at least contains less) pesticides, fertilizers and other chemicals. Many times it is best to get dandelion from your local natural grocer or buy it in tea or capsule form.

In Skin Care: Dandelion can be great at fighting skin infections. Dr. Josh Axe, a well-known public figure who supports natural medicine, says that the milky-white substance that you get on your fingers when you break a dandelion stem is highly alkaline. Surprisingly, it also has germicidal, insecticidal and fungicidal properties. Dr. Axe states you can apply the stem's white sap directly to itchy or irritated skin caused by eczema, ringworm, psoriasis, and other skin infections. The raw plant can help ease the itch and repair the skin.

Detox: Dandelion-root tea has historically been used to improve appetite and ease minor digestive ailments. Dandelion tea balances the natural and beneficial bacteria in the intestines. It clears out waste in the kidneys and has been shown to assist in removing toxins from the liver.

Inflammation: Dandelion contains antioxidants and phytonutrients that reduce inflammation throughout the body, which in turn helps relieve pain and reduce swelling.

Immune System: Dandelion boosts the immune system and fights off unwanted microbes and fungi. Dandelion is also high in antioxidants, fiber, calcium, iron, vitamin A, vitamin C and vitamin K, which are all wonderful nutrients for the body.

Edible: The leaves, flowers, and roots are all edible. My favorite ways to get dandelion into my family's diet is with dandelion root tea or tossing a few dandelion leaves into our salads.

Manage Your Stress

Detoxing is not just about food. Stress and lack of exercise can cause a lot of physical and emotional problems that can show up on your skin and in your overall health. Manage your stress by allowing yourself some "down" time—try a trip to the lake for peace and quiet. Meditative movement, like yoga, is also great for quieting your nervous system. And never underestimate the importance of exercise. When we work out, toxins are released from our bodies. This helps us regain balance and optimize health. Breaking a sweat is particularly important because many toxins will come out through perspiration. Saunas are also beneficial for sweating out impurities.

Use the Breath

Surprisingly, breathing releases a lot of toxins in the body. Some people who suffer from anxiety tend to periodically hold their breath during times of stress. This is hard on the body and affects relaxation. So remember to breathe slowly and deeply whenever you are feeling stressed or anxious.

Try a Lymph-Drainage Massage

Stimulating the lymph system can be extremely helpful when detoxing the body. A slow lymph system can lead to a slower elimination of toxins. See page 35 for more on lymph drainage and how to give yourself a lymph-draining facial.

Wholesome, Raw, Unaltered Food Is Best

If your detox plan includes a shake, skip the synthesized powder if possible. I actually love doing shakes every day. Just one drink gives you so many nutrients that you would not normally consume. If you can, make a shake with all raw foods, as it is more easily absorbed and will only have natural ingredients. If you require extra protein, try adding in a nut butter, seed butter, or some other natural ingredient such as organic maca powder.

Here is a list of superfoods that you may want to consider including in your diet or in a smoothie. These foods are wonderful for the body and help the skin. Choose organic whenever possible.

Apples	Ginger	Pumpkin pulp
Avocado	Green tea	Pumpkin seeds
Barley	Honey	Red wine
Beans	Hot peppers	Spinach
Beets	Kefir	Spirulina
Blueberries	Kelp	Sprouts
Broccoli	Kiwi fruit	Sweet potatoes
Cinnamon	Lentils	Tomatoes
Coconut	Olive oil	Turmeric
Dark chocolate	Onions	Walnuts
Flaxseed	Oranges	Wild salmon
Garlic	Pomegranates	Yogurt

"Then God said, 'Behold, I have given you every plant yielding seed that is on the surface of all the earth, and every tree which has fruit yielding seed; it shall be food for you.'"

Genesis 1:29

I have learned over the last decade to think of food as a way to heal rather than a way to comfort. What we put into our body matters. It can either heal us or hurt us. Even though we hear constant hype about the best and worst foods to eat, what I have found to be true is this: if God made the food, it is good and it can heal you. If we have altered the food in any way, aside from cooking and fermenting, it can hurt you. The way God made it in its purest form—fresh apples from the tree, herbs picked from the garden—is the most healthy for us.

Knowing which ingredients to avoid is also helpful. Below is a handy list of ingredients to avoid. When we avoid toxins, we do not have to detox as much. Additionally, how we feel and our energy level is directly connected to what we ingest. The following food additives and ingredients I have found to be very hard on the body; it is best to avoid them.

- Artificial flavors

- Artificial sweeteners (aspartame, sucrose, sucralose)

- DHT, BHA, BHT, TBHQ preservatives

- Food dyes and artificial colors (Red #3, Blue #2, and so on)

- Genetically modified foods (GMO)

- High-fructose corn syrup (also labeled as HFCS, corn syrup, glucose and fructose)

- Maltodextrin and dextrose

- Monosodium glutamate (MSG)

- Recombinant bovine growth hormone (rBGH)

- Refined oils (monoglycerides, diglycerides, canola oil, cottonseed oil)

Whether we like it or not, our produce is being sprayed and altered for quicker, easier production. Research has shown that buying organic is healthier and contains more nutrients than the mass-produced fruits and vegetables. When possible, buy organic. If you are unable to buy organic, use a safe veggie spray to wash them. You can find a DIY veggie spray on the Green Eyed Grace website: GreenEyedGrace.com/DIY-fruit-vegetable-wash-spray.

Cook with Herbs

Herbs are another great way to bring your body and skin back to health. A few of my favorite herbs for detoxing are turmeric, ginger, cinnamon, dandelion, burdock, and nettle.

Stay Hydrated

Our adult bodies are made up of about 60 percent water. When we are dehydrated, our bodies do not function properly, and we get unpleasant symptoms. The skin is also greatly affected by dehydration. One thing you can do to keep your body well hydrated is to drink a glass of water when you wake up, before coffee or anything else. Make sure to drink water frequently throughout the day as well.

Practice Good Habits

Maintaining a healthy lifestyle will make an occasional detox much easier on the body. There will be less reason to detox if you maintain a healthy body with healthy, everyday habits such as eating healthy meals, exercising, praying, stretching and other suggestions I have listed in this book.

Take a Bath

Epsom salts or mineral salts sprinkled in the tub can also help detox the body. And who can pass up a relaxing hot bath? I try to use quiet bath-time for peaceful prayer, which is a nice mental detox. So put on the classical music and let the salts do their work.

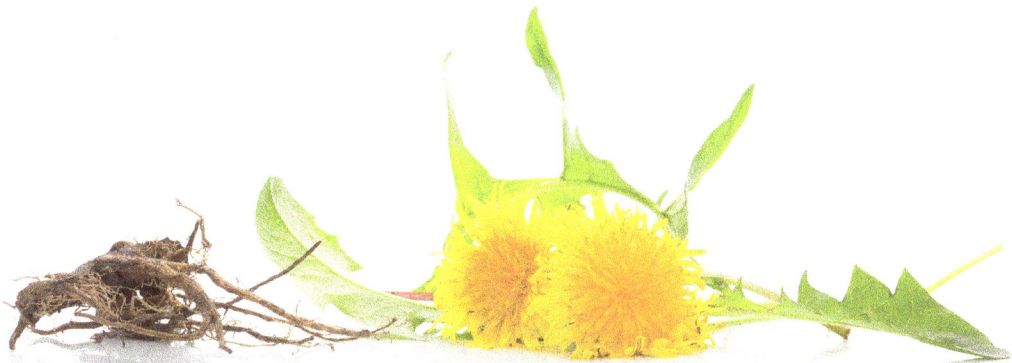

HEALTHY SMOOTHIES & BEVERAGES FOR BEAUTIFUL SKIN

Our skin is a direct reflection of what is happening inside our bodies. Drinking a healthy smoothie is a great trick to give your skin a glow. Berries can help reduce inflammation in our bodies and can reduce puffiness of the skin. Even more important, the ingredients in the Antioxidant-Packed Berry Smoothie recipe (page 191) offer high amounts of vitamins, such as vitamin C, which is highly critical to skin care because it can build and maintain collagen and tissue. Even though vitamin C is often used topically, it is also important to get enough of it through a healthy diet.

Additionally, using yogurt in your smoothies can give you that boost of probiotic (healthy bacteria) that help move food smoothly through your digestive tract. When you have a well-running digestive system, you have a happy body. A happy body means happy skin.

I love using local, raw honey as it can help reduce inflammation and minimize allergy symptoms. Not to mention that a little bit of honey makes anything taste better. Get to know your local beekeepers—ideally the ones whose hives are located among organic fields. You will be amazed at the difference in taste from organically grown honey compared to honey bought in stores. It is delicious!

I went through quite a few recipes before coming up with these beautiful combinations of skin-enhancing beverages. Bring your skin back to life with delicious, antioxidant-packed smoothies, the perfect health drinks that taste great and are good for your body and skin.

Many of the smoothie recipes in the following pages are portioned for "family" size, meaning two adults and two children. Adjust ingredients accordingly for the size batch you prefer. For smoothies, I feel that adults only need six to eight ounces; a child's portion is around four ounces.

ANTIOXIDANT-PACKED BERRY SMOOTHIE

Makes 30 ounces (about 3 smoothies)

1 cup frozen organic blueberries

½ cup frozen organic strawberries

2 ripe bananas

1 cup pure coconut water

½ cup unsweetened almond milk

1 cup ice

1 tablespoon raw, local honey

2 tablespoons plain organic yogurt

I like to use frozen fruits sometimes for convenience and to make an extra-cold batch. However, using fresh fruit is more nutritious.

Blend well and serve immediately.

GREEN-BEAUTY POWER SMOOTHIE

Makes 30 ounces (about 3 smoothies)

4 cups spinach or kale

1 diced cucumber

½ cup water or coconut water

1 lime, juiced

4 carrots, peeled and diced (it's easier if they are cooked)

1 apple, cored and diced

1 cup strawberries

1 cup ice

Blend the greens first. Then add the remaining ingredients and blend until completely smooth. Serve immediately.

GREEN-MONSTER KID'S SMOOTHIE

Makes 30 ounces (about 8 child's-size small smoothies)

This has been a household favorite for many years. I cannot tell you how many recipes I went through before my son accepted a smoothie and drank it all. Now he gets upset if I ever skip his morning shake. Give this one a try for the picky eater/drinker in your house—kid or adult.

3 whole bananas, peeled

½ ripe avocado

1 cup baby spinach, rinsed

1½ cups original almond milk

1 cup coconut water

1 tablespoon pure almond butter*

4 to 5 ice cubes

Additional Add-Ins (optional)

1 teaspoon organic, ground flaxseed

1 tablespoon of raw, organic coconut oil

1 ½ teaspoons raw honey**

1 teaspoon maca powder

Combine all ingredients in a blender. Blend for about 2 minutes or until extra smooth. Serve and enjoy.

* If you have a nut allergy, you can always replace the almond milk with coconut milk or cows milk and the almond butter with sun butter (sunflower seeds) or tahini.

** Children under the age of one should not eat raw honey.

SKIN REPAIR & BALANCE SMOOTHIE

Makes 30 ounces (about 3 smoothies)

1¼ cup organic frozen strawberries*

¼ cup organic frozen blueberries*

1 small clementine orange, peeled and deseeded

½ avocado

4 large slices of organic cucumber

1 tablespoon organic, ground flaxseed

1½ cups coconut water

2 tablespoons almond butter**

2 cups ice

1–2 tablespoons raw, local honey

Combine all ingredients in a blender. Blend until smooth. Serve cold.

You do not have to use frozen berries. I prefer them because it is much more convenient. Fresh is always more nutritious, so it is your preference.

**If you have a nut allergy, substitute sun butter or tahini in place of almond butter.*

HAPPY-SKIN STRAWBERRY SMOOTHIE

Makes 14 ounces (1 large smoothie)

   3/4 cup organic strawberries

   1 tablespoon organic chia seeds

   1 cup organic Greek yogurt

   1 tablespoon raw, unfiltered, local honey

   1/2 cup ice

   1/4 cup pure coconut water

Combine all ingredients in a blender until smooth. Great for a shake "meal" on the go.

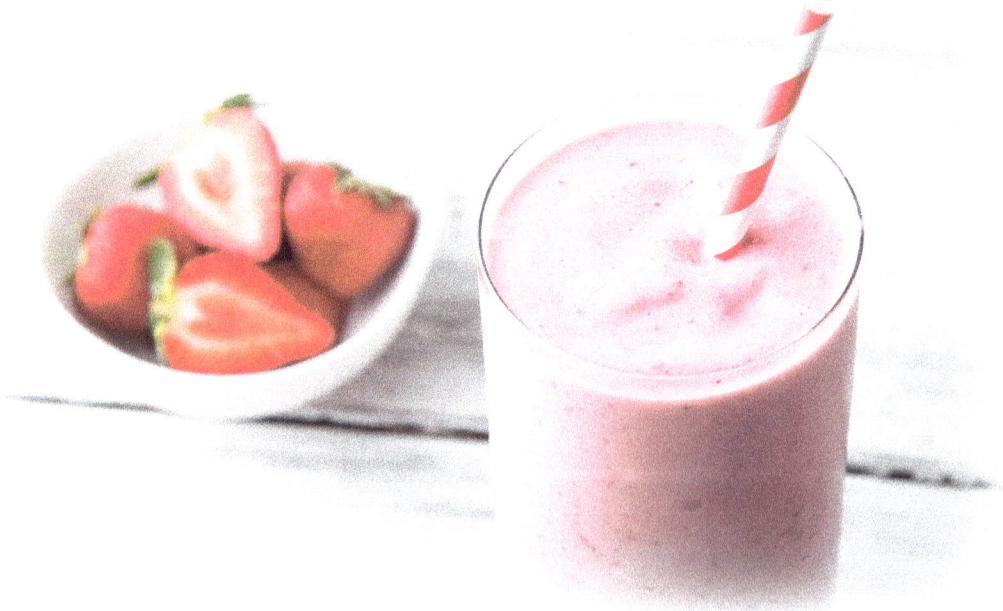

URGENT-REPAIR TEA TONIC

Makes 8 ounces

I like to think of this drink as a non-alcoholic hot toddy. It is great for the body and helps speed up detox and recovery.

> ½–1 teaspoon chopped fresh ginger
>
> 1 teaspoon apple cider vinegar*

Boil 1 cup of water and pour it over the fresh ginger in a mug. Let seep for 4 to 5 minutes. Strain out the ginger. (Alternatively, you can boil the ginger in the water for a couple of minutes and then strain it out.) Once the water has cooled enough to drink, add the apple cider vinegar.

Drink a couple cups of this tea per day when you are feeling under the weather or recovering from sugar and processed food overload.

* To make your own apple cider vinegar, see page 197.

CALM-SOUL SPICED MILK

Makes 8 ounces

This is a wonderful, warm "golden milk" to drink at night before bed. It relieves aches and pains and promotes relaxation. Do not be surprised if you fall asleep on the couch after drinking it.

¾ cup almond milk	1½ teaspoons raw honey
¼ cup coconut water	2 shakes of black pepper
⅛ teaspoon turmeric	2 shakes of cardamom
⅛ teaspoon cinnamon	saffron (just a pinch)

Combine all ingredients in a saucepan. Heat on low heat. Mix well by using a wire whisk to eliminate clumps. Heat for a few minutes to let the saffron absorb into the almond milk. Serve and enjoy.

THE MANY BENEFITS OF
APPLE CIDER VINEGAR

Apple cider vinegar (ACV) has been used for thousands of years. In fact, around 400 BC, Hippocrates, the father of modern medicine, prescribed apple cider vinegar mixed with honey for a variety of ailments, including coughs and colds. Interestingly, a dilution of apple cider vinegar was drank by ancient Persians to keep the body lean. And many health advocates in our current era often claim ACV can help manage weight if a small, diluted amount is consumed each day.

There are other applications as well. For thousands of years, apple cider vinegar has been used to preserve food, and even today it is regarded as a useful, non-toxic cleaning product.

One of my favorite benefits of ACV are that it benefits the skin. When used topically, diluted apple cider vinegar can act as a restorative toner for the skin because its high acidic levels help to balance the skin's pH. It has a long history of cosmetic uses and was frequently used for skin care throughout the ages.

Apple cider vinegar's antiseptic properties can also be used in home remedies for skin conditions that are caused by bacterial overgrowth. In addition, its astringent function can minimize acne breakouts. When used as a hair rinse, ACV can remove heavy residues left behind from soaps and shampoos.

Thankfully, apple cider vinegar is quite simple to make. Often, when making it yourself with organic apples, you get a mild sweet-tasting vinegar that is actually pleasant to drink. In fact, I think it is much more palatable than the vinegar you buy at the store—and homemade ACV makes using it on your skin even more meaningful.

APPLE CIDER VINEGAR

Fermentation time: 4 to 6 weeks

Use this organic vinegar for cooking, cleaning, skin care or as an ingredient in health drinks.

1 Mason jar (clear glass, extra-large size)	Water
	Canning weight
3–5 organic apples	Cheesecloth, coffee filter, or breathable fabric
Pure cane sugar	

Wash the apples, remove the cores and seeds, and chop them into small to medium sized pieces (it is not necessary to peel the apples). Fill an extra-large Mason jar three-quarters full with the chopped apples. Use a measuring cup to add enough water to completely cover the apples—and be sure to keep track of how many cups it takes in order to calculate your sugar amount. Leave a couple of inches of space at the top of the jar. Add 1 tablespoon of sugar per cup of water you used in the jar.

Use a canning weight to keep apples submerged in the water. You do not want apples poking up through the water at the top. Cover the Mason jar with either cheesecloth (use a double layer) or a coffee filter or clean piece of fabric. Secure it with a canning ring. It is important to keep gnats and other insects out of your vinegar, so make sure this is secured well.

Place your vinegar in a warm, dark spot for two weeks. Check on it every couple of days, stirring once in a while with a clean spoon to avoid contamination. Be sure to replace the cover afterwards. A scum may form on top—don't worry, it is part of the fermentation process. Mold, however, is not good. If you notice mold growing on top, you will want to discard your ACV batch and start over.

The scum that develops on top will eventually turn into a scoby also know as the "mother" which is packed with friendly bacteria and gives rise to your ACV. You can remove it or you can just leave it floating in your vinegar.

After two weeks, strain all the apple scraps from the liquid. Discard the scraps and put the liquid back in the jar. Cover the jar again with a clean covering (breathable cloth, coffee filter, cheesecloth) and return to a dark, warm area.

Leave the vinegar for at least two weeks more. I like to leave mine for four weeks to get a stronger apple cider vinegar. After a couple weeks you will notice a strong cider scent. Once you are happy with the smell and taste of the vinegar, use a funnel to pour it into sterilized glass beverage bottles or jars. Cap the bottles and store them in the refrigerator.

When to Discard: Vinegar will keep for months (even years) this way

QUICK RECIPES FOR REFRESHING SPA SIPPERS

Creating your own spa water can add a special touch to any holiday or get-together with friends, and these healthy sippers are even better if you have your own spa party. (For spa party ideas, be sure to read chapter 19.) Below are a couple of refreshing, infused waters that are always a hit. These are also multipurpose, as they can eliminate toxins and reduce inflammation in the body. Your guests will love the taste and want to drink more, which can be very hydrating and beneficial for the skin.

CUCUMBER-LEMON SPA WATER

Makes 64 ounces

A simple, yet perfectly refreshing, infused water. Each cup gives you a little blast of vitamin C and antioxidants.

    8 cups water

    1 medium cucumber, thinly sliced

    1 medium lemon, thinly sliced

    Ice

Combine all ingredients in a large pitcher or a water container with a spout. Let marinate for several hours, refrigerating if possible. I like to keep the cucumber and lemon in the water because it looks pretty, but you can strain it out if you prefer.

When to Discard: about 4 days, refrigerated

STRAWBERRY-MINT SPA WATER

Makes 64 ounces

The subtle taste of fresh strawberries with a crisp aftertaste makes this my favorite spa water. When I serve this light, refreshing water at parties, it disappears pretty quickly. For a special touch, garnish the glasses with strawberries, oranges, or lemons.

   8 cups water

   1 cup sliced strawberries

   1/2 cup fresh mint leaves

   Ice

Combine all ingredients in a large pitcher or a water container with a spout. Let marinate for several hours, refrigerating if possible. I like to keep the strawberries and mint in the water because it looks pretty, but you can strain it out if you prefer.

When to Discard: about 4 days, refrigerated

CHAPTER 19

Create Your

OWN SPA PARTY

The recipes I offer throughout this book can be used and curated for spa parties that are tailored to your guests. The spa party ideas laid out in this chapter can easily be used for daily skin-care treatments. Follow these fun and easy steps according to your desired age group. For instance, the suggestions for the Spa Party for Kids address sensitive young skin, whereas the Teen Spa Party revolves around natural products that help treat acne. I've even created a special Men's Spa Party featuring skin-care recipes that men have used and liked. And, of course, the Adult Spa Party suggestions are a great place for guests to start trying out all-natural recipes they can make at home.

Spa parties can be held in your living room, kitchen, or wherever you have a good spot with ample space for spreading out your products. Each guest should have a comfortable seat with their very own selection of customized products to try. Be sure to have little trays, plates, or even cute paint palettes

Things You May Need

Mirrors for guests
Warm facial towels or wipes (2 for each guest)
Little trays and cups for snacks and drinks
Products:
  *Cleanser
  *Mask
  *Toner
  *Moisturizer
  *Hand scrub
  *Salts for foot soak
Foot-soaking tub and flower petals
Cucumbers for the eyes
Spa robes/wraps and/or head wraps
Bowls for mixing DIY product
Spoons for mixing DIY product
Containers for storing DIY product
Ingredients for DIY
Music
Tablecloth(s)
Plastic for floor if doing foot soaks
Name tags for guests
Goody bags for guests

for each guest; these should be large enough to contain enough product for the guest to experience each step in a skin care routine.

I do advise that you practice making and using the skin-care recipes in advance of the party so there are no unwanted surprises, such as a product that doesn't turn out as expected.

One of the special tools I like to have on hand at spa parties are fan-shaped brushes for applying products to the face. Also make sure to have a hair wrap or hairband for each guest to keep product out of their hair. Having warm, damp towels and/or facial wipes is also important for helping wipe off skin and clean up messes. You can also prepare samples of products for your guests to take with them as parting gifts.

PLANNING A SPA PARTY FOR KIDS

For children's parties, it is best to keep it really simple. In my experience, they really like foot soaks, although most kids refer to them as foot baths. These can be a lot of work for the parent or host because water needs to be heated beforehand—and getting warm water in and out of all the foot bins can be tricky. However, foot baths add a little luxury to the overall experience.

I always have my amazing colleague, Amy, help me when doing a Spa Party for Kids. She has a bright, positive personality and everyone feels engaged when she is the host. Having a host or partner to help when throwing a spa party makes it much more fun and less stressful. (And you have another adult to share in the fun!)

Amy and I put rose petals in the foot-bath water for the kids, and they always think that is amazing! Children really love the little things. Then we massage their hands with lotion while they are soaking their feet—so simple! They all giggle—it is adorable!

My daughter still talks about how much she loves the spa party we had when I was practicing skin recipes on her to find out what worked and what did *not*. I have learned a lot since then. For instance, it is imperative to have your cleanser, lotions, and creams pre-made and ready to apply beforehand. One thing my daughter was not happy with was how difficult it was to remove the facial mask. Kids do not want to mess with complicated products— they feel special just being pampered. My daughter sipped on her special drink while we applied products, and we asked her periodically how she felt, making sure she was relaxed.

At the end of the party, we gave her a little goody bag with a homemade chapstick, a little hand-held mirror, chocolates, and stickers. She was so happy she could not stop smiling and jumping around. She felt so special.

When throwing a kid's spa party, it is easier if you have a small group (three to six children) with an age range from five to eleven years old. Usually, children aged four and under have a very hard time sitting still during the application of products. Sometimes they want to put products in their mouth, be disruptive, and so on. It can be too much work for the parent or host, so if you do want to include a young child in the group, make sure you have a parent who is helping them do everything. That way you can focus on the group as a whole.

With a children's group, it is nice to offer finger foods that are easy to eat and minimally messy: fruit, vegetables and dip, snack crackers, and either cookies without frosting or homemade cake pops for dessert. And if you want to create a "fancy" party atmosphere, I've found that sipping sparkling cider from fancy cups, makes kids feel extra special.

Spa Party for Kids (age 5–11) Choose one or more options in each of the five categories below— or feel free to substitute a different favorite recipe from this book. Mix and match to create the perfect party experience for children.		
Cleansers	Sweet & Gentle Facial Cleanser (page 43)	Hydrating Olive Oil Cleanser (page 41)
Masks	Kid-Friendly Moisturizing Mask (page 71)	Sweet Banana Moisture Mask (page 71)
Moisturizers	Nice & Gentle Skin Oil (page 101)	Lavender Body Butter (page 117)
Body Treatments	Fizzing Bath Truffles (page 113)	Use the Gentle Lavender Bath Salts for Kids for a Foot Bath or DIY (page 112)
Beverages	Green-Monster Kid's Smoothie (page 192)	Strawberry-Mint Spa Water (page 199)

PLANNING A SPA PARTY
FOR TEENAGERS

Doing parties for teens has been the most meaningful spa party experience for me personally. Many teens are struggling with self-image issues and suffer from unwanted, embarrassing acne and breakouts, which is one reason I offer a lot of helpful information throughout the book about clearing up acne.

Talking about pimples can be a sensitive subject, and an easier way to approach the issue is to write the acne-preventing tips from chapter 17 on cards and hand them out to teens. However, if the kids are willing to talk about breakouts, that is fantastic as well! Most teens appreciate information about a skin-care routine and products that might help clear their skin. I like doing different exercises with teens in which we talk about skin care and self-care, and I always point out the connection between taking care of yourself and self-esteem.

For one gathering, I handed out two pieces of paper, each with an outline of a head. I asked the teens to write all the negative thoughts and comments they heard or said to themselves on their bad days inside the first head. Then, inside the second head, they wrote a bunch of positive words and thoughts they hear from loved ones and friends. Together, we all tore up the negative-thoughts head while I explained that those mean, negative words can greatly affect how we feel inside. We *all* were crying that day, but it was such a great experience, even for me. It is easy even for adults to forget to "tear up" and "throw away" the mean words we hear as adults too.

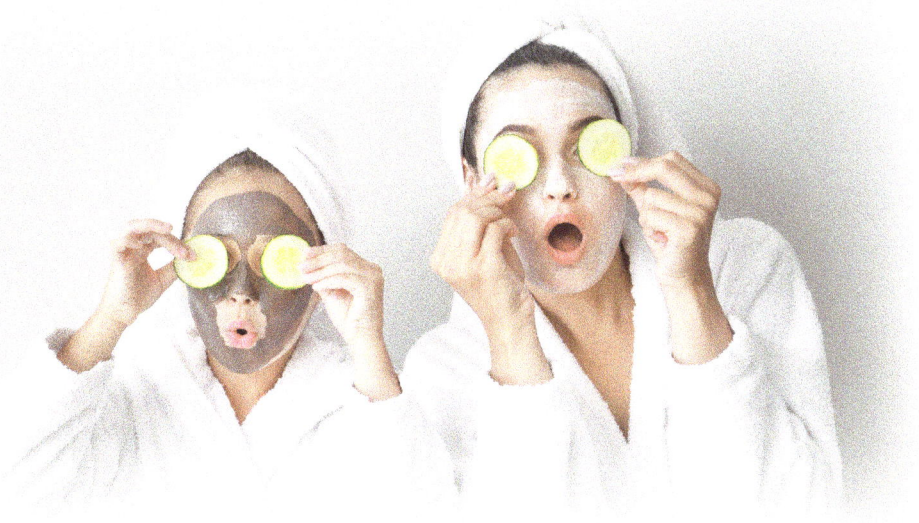

When Amy throws spa parties, she likes to ask her guests questions to keep them engaged. Her favorite question to ask is 'What makes you feel beautiful?' This is a great way to start a conversation about confidence. The younger kids are always eager to answer these types of questions. However, with teens, it takes a little more encouragement. To keep party guests in the conversation, Amy would have a bag of chocolates and reward guests with them when they gave an answer or participated. This really helps to keep the party going!

Anything you can do to make a teen party meaningful is extremely beneficial. A teen party should be approached from a place of love and positive information—not as a way of telling a teen that he/she has not been cleaning his/her face right or making anyone feel bad about their skin. The party should be really fun with interesting products that teens may not normally use. I prefer doing parties for a smaller group of teens, three to six participants. Any more than that, and it is difficult to keep them engaged.

It is nice to serve fancy hors d'oeuvres like chocolate-covered strawberries, fruit kabobs, cucumber sandwiches and pretty cakes. Teens also love sipping sparkling cider from champagne glasses for a glamorous, sophisticated feel. Letting them make one product of their own is really fun too. Sugar scrubs or bath salts are easy to make, and they are a wonderful product that they can make for themselves or as a gift for someone else.

One thing a lot of teens want to know about is skin care routines and how to use products. The handy mix and match chart in this section is a great way to encourage a skin care routine in

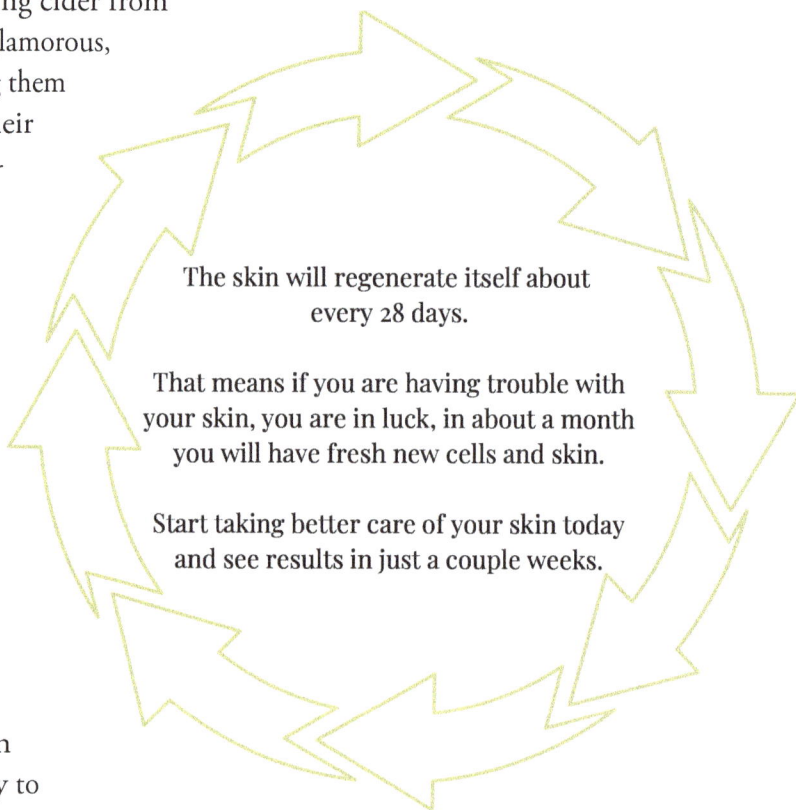

The skin will regenerate itself about every 28 days.

That means if you are having trouble with your skin, you are in luck, in about a month you will have fresh new cells and skin.

Start taking better care of your skin today and see results in just a couple weeks.

How the skin regenerates itself after a breakout

just a couple easy steps. Using the different products that are laid out in the chart below, can help teens get comfortable with products and discover their preferences - deciding what products they may want to keep using in the future.

As a parting gift, I also love to give the "You Are Beautiful" stickers (from You-Are-Beautiful. com) along with a little organic chocolate. This is a simple gesture that makes teenagers feel so special. You can buy a big stack of stickers through this website and hand them out to guests.

Spa Party for Teens (age 12–19) Choose one or more options in each of the six categories below— or feel free to substitute a different favorite recipe from this book. Mix and match to create the perfect party experience for teenagers.		
Cleansers	Honey-Coconut Facial Scrub (page 43)	Gentle Acne Facial Cleanser (page 44)
Masks	Nourishing Turmeric Traditional Mask (page 69)	Activated Charcoal Skin-Clearing Mask (page 73)
Toner & Facial Steam	Acne-Clearing Vanilla Toner (page 48)	Crisp Herbal Facial Steam (page 52)
Moisturizers	Coconut-Vanilla Facial Crème (page 100)	Light Aloe Facial Moisturizer (page 99)
Body Treatments	Coconut-Lemon Sugar Scrub (page 59)	Magnesium-Packed Foot Detox (page 111)
Beverages	Antioxidant-Packed Berry Smoothie (page 191)	Strawberry-Mint Spa Water (page 199)

PLANNING A SPA PARTY FOR ADULTS

There is a pretty wide range of what you can do when throwing an adult spa party. You can host one for mile-marker birthdays or bridal and baby showers. And themes are always fun. For example, if your best friend loves Hawaii, why not choose a beach theme with salt scrubs and tropical drinks?

Usually spa parties for adults—either all women or co-ed gatherings—are more about socializing and spending time together. Making an activity of preparing the DIY products in this book can also be fun, and your guests will feel really pampered, especially if you send them home with a nicely printed recipe card and a pre-labeled glass jar for storing their skin-care products.

To make things easier on yourself as the host, opt for doing a potluck, or ask a couple of your friends to help you organize and buy ingredients for the skin-care recipes you are featuring. Offering some helpful tips on skin care or even doing a skin-care trivia game can be fun and educational. Use the information in this book, and share what you know about a good skin care routine, sun protection or about waxing as a way to inform your guests on different skin-care tips.

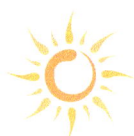

Sun Protection

The sun is responsible for approximately
80% of aging

Stick with zinc oxide or titanium dioxide based sunscreens to physically block out the sun which block out both UVA and UVB rays

The sun is actually GOOD for us, it is the OVEREXPOSURE that is bad

Wear hats, keep to the shade and try not to stay in direct sunlight for long periods

Share tips about sun protection with guests at your adult spa party.

Spa Party for Adults
Choose one or more options in each of the six categories below—
or feel free to substitute a different favorite recipe from this book.
Mix and match to create the perfect adult party experience.

Cleansers	Honey-Coconut Facial Scrub (page 43)	Gentle Acne Facial Cleanser (page 44)
Masks	Chocolate Mud Mask (page 74)	Activated Charcoal Skin-Clearing Mask (page 73)
Toner & Facial Steam	Simple Brightening Lemon Toner (page 47)	Young & Refreshed Facial Steam (page 51)
Moisturizers	Coconut-Vanilla Facial Crème (page 100)	Light Aloe Facial Moisturizer (page 99)
Body Treatments	Lemon-Peppermint Foot Cream (page 119)	Magnesium-Packed Foot Detox (page 111)
Beverages	Green-Beauty Power Smoothie (page 191)	Cucumber-Lemon Spa Water (page 198)

PLANNING A SPA PARTY FOR MEN

I admit that spa parties for guys do not happen that often. Men are usually not as interested in making products or even putting them on their skin, for that matter. However, there are a few guys that absolutely love this stuff and are fascinated with the concept of all-natural DIY skin care. And then, of course, there are those guys who let their wives or girlfriends drag them to these kinds of events and put weird masks and scrubs on their face because they are very supportive of their insistent significant other. [Errr … Cough, cough—Sorry husband!—cough.]

In the next section are suggestions for what products you might start with if you have a male at your Spa Party for Teens or if you have a loved one who is struggling with acne or skin issues who does not know a lot about proper skin-care.

A spa party for guys does not need to be extravagant. It could be as easy as a barbecue with some pampering, but you definitely need to know your audience. If the guy(s) in your life are *not* into this sort of thing, why not simply send them home with a couple of homemade products to try at their leisure? They might end up loving them!

"The progressive development of man is vitally dependent on invention. It is the most important product of his creative brain."

~ Nikola Tesla

Spa Party for Guys (teen/adult) Choose one or more options in each of the six categories below— or substitute different recipes from this book. Mix and match to create the perfect party experience for the men in your life.		
Cleansers	Honey-Coconut Facial Scrub (page 43)	Gentle Acne Facial Cleanser (page 44)
Masks	Brightening Turmeric Glow Mask (page 68)	Activated Charcoal Skin-Clearing Mask (page 73)
Toner & Facial Steam	Acne-Clearing Vanilla Toner (page 48)	Crisp Herbal Facial Steam (page 52)
Moisturizers	Coconut-Vanilla Facial Crème (page 100)	Light Aloe Facial Moisturizer (page 99)
Body Treatments	Lemon-Peppermint Foot Cream (page 119)	Magnesium-Packed Foot Detox (page 111)
Beverages	Antioxidant-Packed Berry Smoothie (page 191)	Strawberry-Mint Spa Water (page 199)

Spa parties can be made super simple or uniquely complex, depending on your time, resources and imagination. There are so many easy skin-care recipes to try, which allows you, the host, to be creative. Whether you decide on a simple party or an extravagant celebration, your guests will leave feeling motivated to take better care of their skin.

GLOSSARY OF SKIN-FRIENDLY INGREDIENTS

Activated charcoal: In skin care, activated charcoal absorbs dirt from the pores and bacteria from blemishes. This helps purify and detoxify the skin. Charcoal masks can be beneficial for oily skin, breakouts, and acne.

"There is the music of Heaven in all things."

~ Saint Hildegard of Bingen

Almond extract: Smells absolutely beautiful in skin care and is nourishing to the skin.

Almond oil: Cold-pressed oil is best. An anti-inflammatory oil that also helps with itchiness and hydration.

Aloe vera: Aloe vera has been used in skin care for centuries. It has a moisturizing, emollient effect on the skin. In addition to skin care, aloe vera can be used as a topical remedy for bug bites, burns, infections, inflammation, and swelling.

Apricot oil: Absorbs very easily and has similar properties to almond oil. It helps minimize fine lines because it is very nourishing and healing to the skin.

Argan oil: Great for healing and protecting the skin. It also hydrates and absorbs nicely.

Avocado and avocado oil: Cold-pressed oil is best. This beneficial oil contains omega-6 fatty acids that nourish the skin. It is high in vitamin B and potassium, which can give your face a glow. Avocado works great as a topical oil, although eating an avocado a day can also give your skin and hair a beautiful glow. So eat them up!

Bananas: Rich in vitamins and minerals, bananas are great for all skin types. They're gentle enough for sensitive skin but effective enough for oily skin. Bananas soften the skin while putting nourishment back into the skin. Very effective in moisturizing dry or sensitive skin.

Beet powder: Beets can stimulate cell reproduction and repair. They are also high in antioxidants, which help to protect the skin from damage from our environment. Topically, beets keep the skin hydrated and glowing.

Bentonite clay: This natural ingredient deeply cleanses your skin, removes toxins and dirt. Helpful for acne and balancing oily skin.

Borage seed oil: This nourishing oil contains high concentrations of gamma-linolenic acid (GLA) and other beneficial fatty acids that calm and sooth dry and/or irritated skin.

Burdock: A skin-soothing antioxidant. Can help ease acne and eczema breakouts. When drank as a tea, burdock is a wonderful detoxifier for blood and the lymph system.

Calendula oil and tincture: Calendula tincture has amazing benefits for the skin. It is most commonly used to reduce inflammation and irritation. Effective at calming acne and hydrating the skin.

Cardamom: This exotic spice contains many compounds that are believed to act as an antioxidant, prevent disease, and promote better health. More important, cardamom is believed to detox the body and alleviate depression.

Carrot seed oil: Full of nutrients such as beta-carotene and vitamins A and E. Calming to the skin; helps reduce itching.

Castor oil: One of my favorite oils to clear up eczema is castor oil. It is thicker in texture and coats the skin well, while still allowing it to breathe. Extremely moisturizing with anti-inflammatory properties.

Chamomile oil and tea: Acts as an anti-inflammatory, and has antibacterial properties for the skin and body. Chamomile tea can also be used as a compress to calm irritated skin.

CALENDULA

Calendula is part of the marigold family. A beautiful, delicate flower, brilliant in yellow or orange and containing many benefits for the skin and body. The calendula flower is commonly found throughout Western Europe, the Mediterranean region, and parts of Southern Asia. However, in Colorado we are more familiar with the French marigold (Tagetes) varieties. These marigolds are a common garden flower, mainly used to ward off insects. They are brightly sprinkled throughout flower gardens to add color and variety. The French marigold is different from calendula (pot marigold), which is described herein.

Calendula is edible and used in a variety of recipes. Most French marigold varieties are not edible and do not possess the same healing properties for skin care. Calendula is a common herbal remedy used in many skin preparations. The common name "marigold" refers to the Virgin Mary. Most likely, it was given this name in the fourteenth century. Marigold was an important ingredient in ancient recipes used in fighting the plague.

One of the most impressive skin-care benefits of calendula is its ability to quickly heal the skin. Calendula can be used for cuts, scrapes, inflammation, circulation, irritation, dryness, skin brightening, and acne.

Chili peppers: Contain capsaicin, which can help desensitize pain receptors. Capsaicin binds to a nerve receptor called VR1, which signals the brain to think you are being exposed to something hot. The nervous system responds by releasing a neurotransmitter called substance P. Once all the substance P in this area is depleted, no more pain signals can travel from that area to the brain. After the heat sensation fades, the sense of pain is significantly reduced. Crushed red pepper, when infused with oil, will give a tingle to the skin and ease tense muscles to offer relief.

Cinnamon: Very beneficial as it brings blood and nutrients to the skin's surface. Cinnamon is a sweet spice that improves the taste of many delicious foods, but it is also great for your skin. Lab studies have found that cinnamon may reduce inflammation, have antioxidant effects, and fight bacteria.

Cocoa butter: Naturally contains beneficial nutrients and antioxidants that can hydrate the skin and minimize fine lines. It is important to buy cocoa butter in its most pure form. Apply right after bathing for best results.

Coconut oil: Raw, unrefined, and fractionated coconut oil can be effective on acne due to its anti-inflammatory properties. ("Fractionated" means the coconut oil has been broken down so it doesn't harden like regular coconut oil.) Applying coconut oil to your skin can improve hydration and is a wonderful replacement for mineral oil. Fractionated coconut oil absorbs quickly into the skin and can help carry a sweet scent. Organic, raw, cold-pressed and unrefined is best. Some swear by organic coconut oil. Its nourishing properties have been known to heal and treat eczema. Having coconut in your regular diet is great for the skin. If you are not able to put it on your skin, try using it in your smoothies and heal from the inside out.

Colloidal silver: One of my favorite ingredients, colloidal silver is an amazing liquid with tiny, suspended particles of silver. It has historically been used to treat bacterial, viral, and fungal infections. **Note:** Not all colloidal silvers are the same. Check the ppm (parts per million). A colloidal silver product with only 30 ppm is not going to be as strong as one that is 150 ppm. The stronger the better when using in skin-care products. If you are considering taking colloidal silver as a supplement, it is important to do extensive research on the effects it can have on the body and what dosage is appropriate.

CoQ10 : Contained in many foods we eat (such as meat, spinach, broccoli, strawberries, and oranges) CoQ10 helps to generate energy. CoQ10 acts as an antioxidant, which protects cells from damage. Thankfully, this nutrient occurs naturally in the body but diminishes as we age.

Dandelion: Dandelion can be great at fighting skin infections. It has germicidal, insecticidal, and fungicidal properties. You can also use the white sap of a dandelion's highly alkaline stem and apply it directly to itchy or irritated skin caused by eczema, ringworm, psoriasis, and other skin infections. The raw plant can help ease the itch and repair the skin. Dandelion tea also aids in liver detox for the body.

Diatomaceous earth: Diatomaceous earth (DTE) is almost entirely made of silica, which can help promote stronger hair, skin, and nails. Be sure to use food-grade DTE rather than the type garden-ers use to eliminate unwanted bugs on their produce. Non food-grade diatomaceous earth is often mixed with chemicals for outdoor use. DTE can cleanse the digestive tract when taken internally and supports healthy digestion. Topically it works wonderfully as an exfoliant and detox mask.

Epsom salts: Epsom salts are crystals of hydrated magnesium sulfate used for sore muscles, body aches, laxatives, or medical use. Magnesium flakes (or salts) are magnesium chloride. Even though Epsom salts are a form of magnesium, the magnesium flakes have a different molecular structure.

Essential oils: Almost everyone is familiar with essential oils these days, but we explore the benefits of certain oils throughout this book. Each essential oil carries its own benefits. Use sparingly and do not ingest.

Evening primrose oil: Can be very healing for dry skin. Helps with skin repair, inflammation, and irritation. Mostly sold in capsule form. Break and apply directly to skin or mix with a carrier oil.

Ginger: In skin care, ginger can promote blood circulation, calm acne and help sore muscles, aches and pains. Packed with antioxidants, it can also provide smoother skin and give a radiant glow.

Glycerin (vegetable, food grade): A clear, odorless, thick liquid made from certain plant oils such as palm, soy and/or coconut oil. Vegetable glycerin is made by heating triglyceride-rich vegetable fats under pressure or together with a strong alkali, such as lye. Then the glycerin splits away from the fatty acids and binds with water. This thick, syrup-like liquid comes in very handy in thickening products and/or helping the skin absorb products.

Grapeseed oil: Grapeseed oil may not have as many healing properties as the other oils listed above. However, it penetrates the skin very well, which allows the other oils to do their job. Grapeseed oil is a very mild oil and great for sensitive skin.

Green tea: Contains polyphenols that help to reduce acne and calms the overproduction of the skin's natural oils. A natural anti-inflammatory that can help prevent UV damage, green tea is rich in antioxidants that protect the skin and body when drank as a tea or applied topically.

Himalayan salt: Himalayan salt is a red rock salt mined in Pakistan. The red rock salt contains large amounts of natural minerals that the body loves. Soaking in these salts can help balance the body's pH levels and aid in detoxification.

Honey: Honey firms the skin and smoothes fine lines. It can also relieve dry skin, balance combi-nation skin and clear up breakouts.

Jojoba oil: Jojoba oil closely resembles human sebum, the oil naturally produced by skin. It is effective for all skin types. Extremely moisturizing, nourishing, and therapeutic for the skin. Can be used as a carrier oil when applying essential oils directly to the skin. It may seem a little greasy, but jojoba absorbs well and helps balance skin.

A WORD ABOUT LAVENDER

Lavender has more than forty different types of species. Lavender (Lavandula genus) is a widely known herb that was used even in biblical times. Some considered it a holy herb. In the past it was often used as a perfume because of its light, pretty scent – it was frequently used to refresh clothes and hair.

In current times, it is mostly used for its calming properties. Lavender promotes relaxation and is a pleasant scent to lift the mood. It also can be extremely beneficial in wound care.

Many parents love it for its ability to ease pain caused by cuts, scrapes, and burns and to heal wounds. It is gentle enough to use on children. Lavender is also said to be good for psoriasis and other skin problems making it a favorite among professionals.

Lavender flowers: Lavender can be very soothing to the skin and calming to the nerves. Used in biblical times as a deodorizer and healing agent.

Lemon juice: One hundred percent pure lemon juice can lighten dark spots on the skin. Lemons have antibacterial properties, which help reduce acne. Lemon juice can get deep into the pores to give you cleaner, healthier looking skin.

Magnesium chloride (magnesium flakes): Magnesium chloride is able to be absorbed into the body much easier than Epsom salts (magnesium sulfate), making the effects much more intense. It also aids in detoxifying the body and relaxing tense muscles.

Mango butter: Mango butter is made from the seeds of the mango, and its properties are different from that of straight mango. Mango butter can be very beneficial for the skin. Avoid using straight mango when making your own skin-care products. Mango skin contains bits of the same toxic substance that is in poison ivy and can cause skin irritation. However, eating mango is great for the skin as it is packed with vitamins A and C, and antioxidants.

Neem oil: Produced from the seed of the tropical neem tree, or *Azadirachta indica*, neem oil has been used to treat many conditions over centuries. Known for its strong odor, it is rich in nutrients and used in a variety of beauty products. Can be used as an effective, natural insect repellent as well.

Nettle: Contains natural antioxidants and acts as an anti-inflammatory, astringent, and deodorizer. Nettle can be slightly stimulating in skin care, bringing blood flow to the surface. Nettle tea is a gentle diuretic that aids in flushing waste through the kidneys and assist with seasonal allergies. A very small percentage of people experience side effects after using nettle, also known as stinging nettle. As a precaution, as with any new herb, use a small amount until you know how your body will respond.

Oats: Oats calm and protect the skin. Packed with nutrients to help ease irritated skin. A wonderful, gentle exfoliant.

Olive oil: A moisturizing oil with antibacterial properties. Packed with antioxidants to protect and hydrate the skin.

Orange extract: Smells amazing in skin-care products and is all natural. Helps to even out skin tone and ease acne.

ALL ABOUT OATS

When farmers began planting wheat and barley, they did not care much for oats. They thought of oats as an annoying weed that was always getting into their wheat and barley. During the Bronze Age (3000–1200 BC), farmers in northern Europe began to farm oats on high hilltops where it was too cold for wheat.

Because oats do not contain gluten, they were not helpful for making bread, but many people used oats to make oatmeal or to thicken soup. Oats were also used to feed livestock. Slowly, oats become popular and are now used as an ingredient in many breakfast dishes and desserts.

One of the great benefits of using topical oats is their ability to calm and protect the skin. Oats are rich in omega-3 fatty acids, folate, and potassium. Just as they are nutritious to eat, they also benefit the skin. Oats can ease skin rashes, dermatitis, insect bites, and eczema. Turn a bath into a skin treatment by simply adding a little ground oatmeal. You can also place 1 cup of oatmeal in a cloth bag and add it to your bathwater if you do not want individual bits floating in the water. Either method will ease skin irritation and discomfort.

The gritty texture of ground oats makes it an excellent exfoliator, which removes unnecessary dead skin cells. Ground oats are also a great addition to skin-care masks, which can be beneficial in a skin care routine.

Peppermint leaves: Dried peppermint leaves are used commonly in tea to ease stomach trouble and decongestion. Peppermint extract is also nice on the skin. Refreshing and revitalizing for dull, lifeless skin.

Pineapple: High in vitamin C and bromelain. Bromelain is an enzyme that can soften skin and help with inflammation.

Pomegranate: High in antioxidants and vitamin C. Pomegranate has natural anti-aging properties, reducing wrinkles and fine lines.

Pumpkin: Packed with vitamins A and C, pumpkin has natural anti-aging and antioxidant properties. It also hydrates and softens skin.

Rooibos: Also known as "red bush," rooibos is most commonly used as a tea. Hypoallergenic and antibacterial, which makes it a perfect ingredient for skin-care products.

Rosehip seed oil: An amazing oil that has been used for centuries. It helps with scarring and eczema and is a great source of retinoic acid that can help with fine lines and wrinkles. Pure, organic rosehip oil can be very pricey, so use it in a facial serum or for spot treatment.

Rum: An alcohol that helps carry a sweet scent in products and acts as an antibacterial ingredient.

Safflower oil: Similar to sunflower oil. Soothes rough skin and helps improve the skin's texture.

Saffron: The most expensive spice and for good reason. These deep-colored saffron "threads" come from the purple crocus flower. The threads contain a very high concentration of manganese. Manganese helps regulate blood sugar, metabolize carbohydrates and absorb calcium. Fortunately, a little saffron goes a long way. It is a spice to be added one thread at a time. Just a thread or two can flavor and color an entire pot of rice. Saffron has been used medicinally to calm nerves and to reduce fevers, cramps, and enlarged livers. It has also been used externally for bruises, rheumatism and neuralgia. Saffron is a powerful antioxidant. It is believed to help prevent disease, detox the body, act as a pain reliever, antidepressant, sleep aid and provide radiant skin.

Sage: A strong antibacterial ingredient that can purify the skin by acting as an astringent. Helps to balance oily or troubled skin.

Sea buckthorn oil: Can heal skin injuries such as eczema and minor cuts, scrapes and irritation. Can be very expensive, so mix this oil with a cheaper one, like sunflower, to make it go further.

Sesame oil: Surprisingly this commonly used Asian food oil has a lot of nutrients in it. Helps with skin softening, rich in vitamins and is easy on the skin. It does have a stronger scent, so smell it before applying to make sure you enjoy the scent.

Sugar: Both white and brown sugar make wonderful, sweet smelling, natural exfoliants.

Sunflower oil: A mild and universal oil that contains important peptides, which may help with collagen building. Very helpful at repairing skin cells.

Turmeric: The anti-inflammatory and antioxidant properties of turmeric are both important to treat skin conditions. For acne, using facial masks that contain turmeric can calm blemishes and heal the skin. For eczema, turmeric can reduce inflammation and redness. Contains compounds known as curcuminoids, the most important of which is curcumin, which has been proven to have medicinal properties. Curcumin is the main active ingredient in turmeric. It has powerful anti-inflammatory effects and is a very strong antioxidant. However, it is tough for the body to absorb when ingested. Surprisingly, black pepper assists with absorption, which is why you will often see pepper in recipes with turmeric. Its roots and leaves have long been used in traditional Indian and Chinese medicines for their demonstrated anti-inflammatory, painkilling, antioxidant and anti-cancer properties. Turmeric is used for a variety of ailments including relaxation, pain, stomach trouble and colds. But as you can see from the recipe on page 69, it is also great for the skin.

Vanilla extract Smells amazing, and is nourishing to the skin. Vanilla bean is an anti-inflammatory that smooths and calms the skin, giving it a youthful appearance.

Vodka: An alcohol that helps carry a scent in products. Also acts as an antibacterial ingredient.

Witch hazel: Witch hazel is actually a shrub that acts as a natural astringent. The leaf, bark and twigs are used in a distillery process, which gives us the amazing witch hazel astringent found in stores. You can typically purchase witch hazel at a supermarket or a natural grocery store.

Yogurt: Contains lactic acid which helps even out skin tone and sloughs off dead skin cells, helping with skin turnover.

A GUIDE TO SYNTHETIC INGREDIENTS

So many products contain synthetic or chemical ingredients. Even natural and organic body-care products contain a small amount of preservatives in order to extend shelf life. Here is a general reference for some common ingredients that may be lurking in your health and beauty products.

Many of these ingredients are considered toxic to the body. However, the general definitions may be confusing. For that reason I am including a few explanations.

Concern	Definition
Allergen	The substance can cause an allergy to develop or occur.
Bioaccumulation	The gradual accumulation of a substance that can affect the organs and/or cells in the body.
Endocrine disrupter	Substance can affect the hormonal systems and may ultimately lead to cancer, tumors, birth defects, and developmental disorders
Environmental toxin	Toxic substance(s) found in our environment, such as in our air and water.
Respiratory toxin or disrupter	Substance can affect the lungs, breathing, and possibly cause future problems to the lung area.
Organ-system toxicity	Various bodily organs can be negatively affected with repeated exposure to toxins.
Neurotoxicity	Substance can have a negative effect on the brain and nervous systems
Skin, eye or lung irritation	Overexposure, inhalation, or any kind of irritation-type reaction can occur from a substance such as an airborne chemical or other irritant.

The following glossary of synthetic ingredients reflects my personal research and also information from Environmental Working Group's "Skin Deep" website: EWG.org/skindeep. However, I highly encourage you to do your own research if you are concerned about the safety of an ingredient. Being your own advocate is so important for your health.

A

Acrylic acid: Synthetic polymer used as a binder. Can cause organ-system toxicity and/or skin, eye, or lung irritation.

Aluminum: (Aluminum chlorohydrate, aluminum zirconium tetrachlorohydrex, or any aluminum compounds.) Very common in deodorant and is easily absorbed into the skin. Nose and lung irritant, endocrine disrupter, neurotoxicity, organ-system toxicity.

Aluminum oxide: Anti-caking agent. Nose and lung irritant, endocrine disrupter, neurotoxicity, organ-system toxicity.

Ammonium laureth sulfate: A surfactant (a compound that lowers the surface tension of water, thereby making a product glide better and blend better with oil) that contains PEG (polyethylene glycol). Can cause lung, eye and skin irritation. May be contaminated with other manufacturing impurities.

Ammonium persulfate: Inorganic salts used as a lightening agent. Lung, eye and skin irritant, allergen, organ-system toxicity, environmental toxicant.

Amodimethicone: Silicone-based polymer. Some debate on safety, rated as a low concern by Environmental Working Group.

Amyl acetate: Mixed isomers of amyl alcohol. Lung, eye and skin irritant.

B

Benzalkonium chloride: Preservative. Allergen, strong lung, eye and skin irritant.

Benzyl alcohol: Synthetic ingredient used for viscosity and fragrance. Organ-system toxicity, allergen.

Boric acid: Inorganic acid. Endocrine disrupter, organ-system toxicity, skin irritant. Is restricted in other countries.

Bronopol (2-bromo-2-nitropropane-1,3-diol): Antibacterial, preservative. Strong lung, eye and skin irritant, endocrine disrupter, organ-system toxicity, chemical release concerns.

Butylated hydroxyanisole (BHA): Carcinogenic. Preservative and stabilizer, endocrine disrupter, organ-system toxicity.

Butylated hydroxytoluene (BHT): Preservative. Respiratory disrupter, lung, eye and skin irritant, organ-system toxicity.

Butylene glycol: Organic alcohol. Lung, eye and skin irritant.

Butylparaben: Preservative in the paraben family. Eye and skin irritant, endocrine disruptor, environmental contaminant.

C

Ceteareth: (with any numeral following it) Skin absorption enhancer, lung, eye and skin irritant, may be contaminated with other manufacturing impurities.

Cetrimonium chloride: Preservative, skin irritant, environmental toxin.

Cetrimonium bromide: Ammonium compound, preservative. Skin irritant and environmental toxin.

Cetyl alcohol: Organic alcohol, possible organ-system toxicity, environmental toxin.

Citric acid: Naturally occurring citric acid is found in oranges and lemons. Citric acid is an antioxidant and also a natural preservative. Often used in the food industry to add a sour taste to drinks and foods. Possible organ-system toxicity and possible skin irritant.

Chloroacetamide: Preservative. Lung, eye and skin irritant. Toxic if inhaled.

Coal tar: Byproduct of coal used to treat itching. Carcinogen, organ-system toxicity, respiratory irritant, lung and skin irritant. Restricted in many countries.

Cocamide DEA: A chemically modified form of coconut oil, foaming agent. Strong system toxicity, possibly carcinogenic, skin irritant.

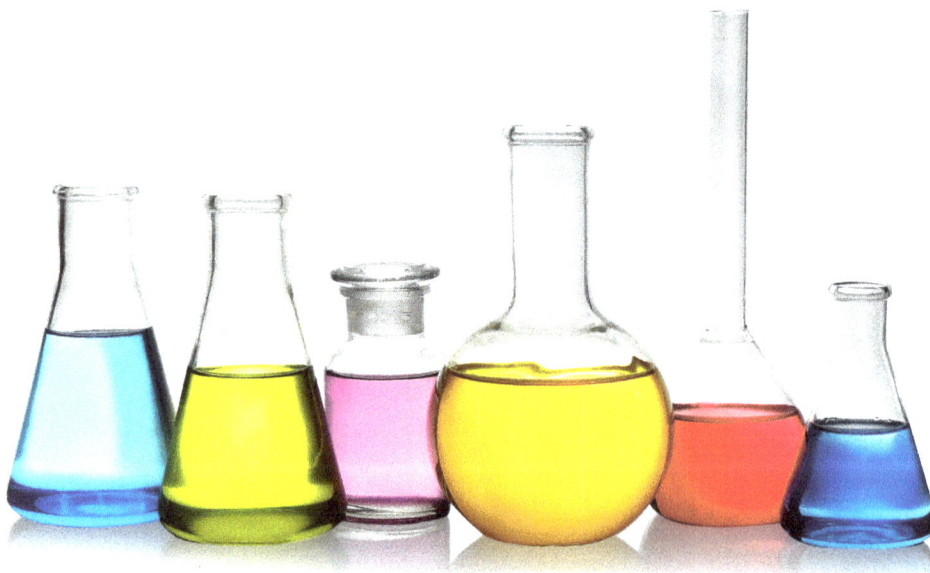

D

D&C Orange 5: Synthetic dye from coal tar or petroleum. Organ-system toxicity, environmental concern.

D&C Red 30 Lake: Synthetic dye. Organ-system toxicity, environmental toxin.

D&C Violet 2: Synthetic dye made from petroleum or coal tar. Organ-system toxicity, environmental toxin.

Dibutyl phthalate: Fragrance, solvent. Neurotoxin, strong endocrine disrupter, organ-system toxicity, environmental toxin, respiratory toxin, restricted in other countries.

Diethanolamine (DEA): Acts as a pH adjuster. Strong lung, eye and skin irritant, organ-system toxicity, possibly carcinogenic. May be contaminated with other manufacturing impurities.

Dimeticone (dimethicone): Silicon-based polymer, skin lubricant, emollient, petroleum derivative. Organ-system toxicity and environmental toxin.

DMDM hydantoin: Formaldehyde releaser, preservative. Possible cancer concern. Lung, eye and skin irritant, allergy and environmental toxin.

E

Ethylparaben: Paraben-family preservative. Skin and eye irritant, endocrine disruptor, environmental contaminant.

Eugenol: Scent chemical found in clove oil, can be manufactured synthetically. Organ-system toxicity and immune-system toxin.

F

FD&C Blue 1: Synthetic dye from petroleum. Organ-system toxicity.

FD&C Green 3: Chemical triphenylmethane dye or color. Eye irritant.

FD&C Yellow 23 (tartrazine): Chemical colorant. Organ-system toxicity, can bioaccumulate in organs and cause allergic reactions.

FD&C Yellow 6: Synthetic dye produced from petroleum. Organ-system toxicity and environmental toxicant.

Formaldehyde: Used in a wide range of cosmetics as a preservative. Known to be carcinogen. Organ-system toxicity, lung, eye and skin irritant, environmental toxin and respiratory irritant. Restricted in other countries.

Formaldehyde resin: Synthetic polymers obtained by the reaction of phenol with formaldehyde. Organ-system toxicity, lung, eye and skin irritant, respiratory irritant, environmental toxin.

Fragrance: Fragrance is not well regulated, so any number of chemical-type ingredients could be included that could be harmful to your health. Possible skin irritant, respiratory irritant, allergen.

G

Glyceryl stearate: Surfactant, emulsifying agent. Low risk, mild toxicity.

Glycolic acid: Used as alpha hydroxy acid in chemical peels and products. Lung, eye and skin irritant.

H

Hyaluronic acid: Naturally present in the human body, found mostly in the eyes and joints. Often hyaluronic acid is extracted from rooster's combs or made by bacteria in the laboratory. Possible organ-system toxicity and possible environmental toxin.

Hydroquinone: Aromatic compound used as topical skin-lightening agent. Organ-system toxicity, skin irritant and allergen, respiratory irritant, environmental toxin.

I

Iodopropynyl butylcarbamate: Preservative. Organ-system toxicity, allergen, respiratory irritant, environmental toxin.

Imidazolidinyl urea: Antimicrobial preservative that functions by forming formaldehyde in cosmetics. Strong skin irritant, can be toxic to the immune system. Environmental concern.

Isobutylparaben: Paraben-family preservative. Strong endocrine disrupter, organ-system toxicity, skin and eye irritant. Can have bioaccumulation in organs causing allergies. Environmental toxin.

Isopropyl stearate: A compound made from alcohol and stearic acid. Acts as a skin-softening agent and emollient in cosmetics. Lung, eye and skin irritant.

L

Lactic acid: Bacterial milk fermentation used as an exfoliant. Possible lung, eye and skin irritant.

Lead acetate: Inorganic salt, hair colorant. Organ-system toxicity, bioaccumulation in organs, human development and reproductive toxin, environmental toxin.

Lecithin: Naturally occurring lipid found in both plants and animals that is used as an emollient and skin conditioner. Possible respiratory irritant.

M

Malic acid: Naturally occurring organic acid. Lung, eye and skin irritant.

Manganese sulfate: Inorganic salt. Organ-system toxicity, environmental toxin.

Methylparaben: Paraben-family preservative. Endocrine disrupter, immune system toxicant, biochemical/cellular concern.

Mineral oil: Byproduct of petroleum. Organ-system toxicity, possibly carcinogenic.

Methylchloroisothiazolinone/methylisothiazolinone: Preservative. Lung, eye and skin irritant, neurotoxin, immune system toxin.

Methylsulfonylmethane (MSM): Organic sulfur compound found in fruit, vegetables, milk, and grains. MSM helps to repair the skin. Possible eye and skin irritation.

Monoethanolamine (MEA)/ethanolamine (ETA): Buffering agent. Organ-system toxicity, lung, eye and skin irritant.

N

Nonoxynol: Emulsifying agent. Bioaccumulation in organs, can be contaminated with other manufacturing impurities.

O

Octoxynol (9, 10, 11, 13, 40): Surfactant, emulsifying agent. Lung, eye and skin irritant, possible organ toxicity, possible environmental toxin. Can be contaminated with other manufacturing impurities.

Oxybenzone (benzophenone): Sunscreen ingredient. Endocrine disrupter, bioaccumulation in cells, biochemical and cellular concerns.

P

P-phenylenediamine: Hair colorant. Organ-system toxicity, lung, eye and skin irritant, environmental toxin.

Padimate O (PABA): Derivative of PABA sunscreen ingredient. Endocrine disrupter, bioaccumulation in cells, biochemical and cellular concerns, environmental toxin.

Parabens: (methyl, ethyl, propyl, benzyl and butyl) Paraben-family preservatives. Endocrine disrupter, immune system toxicant, biochemical/cellular concern.

Paraffin: (paraffinum liquidum, paraffin petrolatum) Petroleum-based skin conditioner. Organ-system toxicity.

PEG-100 stearate (stearic acid): Organ-system toxicity, environmental toxin. May be contaminated with other manufacturing impurities.

Petrolatum: (soft paraffin, white petrolatum, petroleum jelly) Petroleum-based skin conditioner. Organ-system toxicity. May be contaminated with other manufacturing impurities.

Phenol: Added to deodorant, exfoliants, fragrances and/or added as a preservative. Organ-system toxicity, bioaccumulation in cells, lung, eye and skin irritant. Restricted in other countries.

Phenoxyethanol: Preservative. Organ-system toxicity, lung, eye and skin irritant.

Phthalate: Plastic softener common in cosmetics. Helps lotions penetrate and soften skin. Organ-system toxicity, bioaccumulation in cells, environmental toxin.

Polyethylene glycol (PEG): (also labeled as "steareths" and "propylene glycol") Emulsifying agent. Organ-system toxicity. May be contaminated with other manufacturing impurities.

Polyethylene terephthalate: Viscosity ingredient. Organ-system toxicity.

Polysorbate 20: Emulsifying agent. Organ-system toxicity. May be contaminated with other manufacturing impurities.

Polysorbate 80: Emulsifying agent. Organ-system toxicity. May be contaminated with other manufacturing impurities.

Potassium persulfate: Inorganic salt, oxidizing agent. Organ-system toxicity, lung, eye and skin irritant.

Propyl acetate: Synthetic solvent, fragrance ingredient. Organ-system toxicity, lung, eye and skin irritant.

Propylene glycol (PG): Organic alcohol, skin-conditioning agent. Organ-system toxicity, lung, eye and skin irritant.

Propylparaben: Paraben-family preservative. Endocrine disrupter, immune system toxicant, biochemical/cellular concern.

R

Resorcinol (m-hydroquinone, 1,3-benzenediol): Bleaching agent. Endocrine disrupter, organ-system toxicity, lung, eye and skin irritant, environmental toxin.

S

Silica: Most common source is fine sand. Anticaking agent, exfoliant. Organ-system toxicity if airborne, bioaccumulation if airborne.

Sodium metabisulfite: Preservative. Lung, eye and skin irritant, organ-system toxin, allergen.

Sodium laureth/lauryl sulfate: Cleansing agent, emulsifier. Organ-system toxicity, lung, eye and skin irritant. May be contaminated with manufacturing impurities.

T

Tartaric acid: Organic acid, pH adjuster, fragrance. Low risk of toxicity.

Teflon (PTFE/tetrafluoroethylene): This nonstick coating used in cookware once contained a compound known as PFOA, which raised health concerns. Most Teflon-coated products no longer contain this compound, which has been exchanged for PTFE, which has not been known to have as many health concerns as PFOA. PTFE is also used as a skin conditioner to help products glide on better. May be contaminated with other manufacturing impurities, lung irritant.

Tetrasodium EDTA: Chelating agent. Absorbs quickly into the skin, but has a low risk of toxicity.

Thimerosal (thiomersal): Mercury-based preservative. Organ-system toxicity, neurotoxin, endocrine disrupter, environmental toxin. May be contaminated with other manufacturing impurities.

Thioglycolic acid: Organic acid, exfoliant. Organ-system toxicity, strong skin irritant. May be contaminated with other manufacturing impurities.

Toluene (methylbenzene): Solvent. Organ-system toxicity, human development toxicant, respiratory toxin, lung, eye and skin irritant, bioaccumulation, environmental toxin.

Triclosan: Antibacterial and antifungal agent. Organ-system toxicity, endocrine disrupter, lung, eye and skin irritant, bioaccumulation, allergen, environmental toxin. May be contaminated with other manufacturing impurities.

Triethanolamine: Surfactant, emulsifier. Organ-system toxicity, allergen. May be contaminated with other manufacturing impurities.

Triphenyl phosphate: Plasticizer. Endocrine disrupter, neurotoxin, environmental toxin.

RESOURCES

Dr. Josh Axe, DC, DNM, CNS Dr. Axe is a well-known doctor of chiropractic and natural medicine. His website offers lots of information about food, diet, and the latest health trends: DrAxe.com.

Campaign for Safe Cosmetics An organization that works to protect consumers from harmful chemicals linked to health issues and cancer: www.SafeCosmetics.org

"Collaborative on Health and the Environment's Toxicant and Disease Database" This searchable database summarizes links between contaminants and their effects on the human body: www.HealthAndEnvironment.org.

The Complete Illustrated Holistic Herbal by David Hoffman (Rockport, MA: Element Books), 1999.

"Cosmetic Ingredient Hotlist: Prohibited and Restricted Ingredients in Canada" www. Canada.ca/en/health-canada/services/consumer-product-safety/cosmetics/cosmetic-ingredient-hotlist-prohibited-restricted-ingredients.html

Cosmetic Ingredient Review A website that reviews the safety of ingredients used in cosmetics. www.CIRsafety.org

Environmental Working Group's Skin Deep A wonderful resource for checking ingredient information when preparing products or when purchasing certain ingredients: www.EWG.org/skindeep

The Essential Oil Company A great website to buy ingredients and supplies for DIY recipes: www.EssentialOil.com

Hildegard Von Bingen's Physica: The Complete English Translation of Her Classic Work on Health and Healing, translated by Priscilla Throop (Rochester, VT: Healing Arts Press, 1998.

The Holy Bible, King James and ESV versions. I love the biblical resources available through the online version of The Holy Bible. There's a phone app to help you read or listen to the Word anywhere you go. The website is also extremely helpful: www.bible.com

International Agency for Research on Cancer (IARC) A website that focuses on worldwide collaborative research on cancer: www.IARC.fr

Milady's Standard Fundamentals for Estheticians, Ninth Edition by Joel Gerson, et. al., (Thomson Delmar Learning), 2004.

Mind Body Green A website that looks at overall wellness with helpful articles and information for many different topics: www.MindBodyGreen.com

The Modern Herbal Dispensatory: A Medicine-Making Guide by Thomas Easley and Steven Horne (Berkeley, CA: North Atlantic Books), 2016.

Mountain Rose Herbs A favorite website for purchasing organic essential oils, supplies, and ingredients. There are also many blog posts and articles about ingredients and more recipes to try: www.MountainRoseHerbs.com

Scorecard The Pollution Information Site is packed with info about toxicants in the air, water, and manufactured products: Scorecard.goodguide.com

U.S. Environmental Protection Agency (EPA) www.EPA.gov

INDEX

ABOUT THE AUTHOR

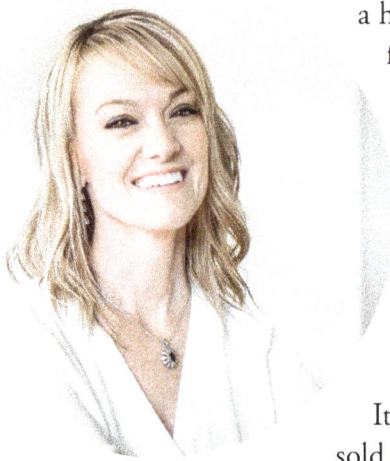

Bethel Jiricek was a former trial paralegal before discovering her true passion. Now she is a mother of four, a certified herbalist and a holistically inspired esthetician. She once struggled to find a chemical-free cream to help with her son's eczema and took matters into her own hands, experimenting with approximately a hundred or so different recipes before she found one that soothed his regular breakouts. As a result, Bethel channeled her passion for effective, natural products into the creation of affordable skin care that contains better ingredients. Today, that passion is known as Green Eyed Grace professional skin care (www.GreenEyedGrace.com). Its comprehensive line of pure, all-natural products are sold in Northern Colorado boutiques as well as at Bethel's spa, Natural Elements Skin Spa, located in Greeley, Colorado.

Bethel knows what it is like to struggle to afford better products for yourself and your family, which is why she wrote this do-it-yourself book. Many years of hard work and determination went into perfecting these recipes and remedies. It is with much love and joy that they are shared with all of you.

"Let all that you do be done in love."

1 Corinthians 16:14

www.ingramcontent.com/pod-product-compliance
Lightning Source LLC
Chambersburg PA
CBHW042349030426
42336CB00025B/3422